INTRODUCTION TO OCCUPATIONAL EPIDEMIOLOGY

Sven Hernberg

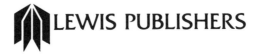

LEWIS PUBLISHERS

Library of Congress Cataloging-in-Publication Data

Hernberg, Sven.
    Introduction to occupational epidemiology / Sven Hernberg.
       p.   cm.
    Includes bibliographical references and index.
    ISBN 0-87371-636-1
    1. Occupational diseases--Epidemiology.   I. Title.
    [DNLM: 1. Epidemiologic Methods.   2. Occupational Diseases-
-epidemiology.   WA 950 H557i]
    RC964.H45   1991
    616.9'803--dc20
    DNLM/DLC
    for Library of Congress   91-41009
                                                           CIP

PRINTED IN THE UNITED STATES OF AMERICA
3 4 5 6 7 8 9 0

Printed on acid-free paper

Preface

Epidemiology has been called the parent discipline of public health. Much of the knowledge of modern occupational medicine also derives from epidemiologic studies. This is especially true for those work-related disorders that are not considered classical occupational diseases. Such diseases are characterized by a multifactorial etiology and their manifestations may be indistinguishable from those of general diseases. For example, a back disorder due to heavy physical work does not differ clinically from a similar disorder brought about by sports injuries or some other causes. Likewise, a lung cancer mainly caused by exposure to nickel salts is indistinguishable from one caused, for example, by cigarette smoking. *Individual* etiologic diagnosis is therefore not possible. Only by studying *groups* of people can the etiologic share of different factors, among them occupational factors, be identified and quantified. There are also many nonspecific syndromes or symptoms that can be induced, to a greater or lesser extent, by occupational factors. These include bronchitis, headache, fatigue, dysfunctions of peripheral nerves, and so forth. Studying the etiology of such manifestations of morbidity also requires an epidemiologic approach.

Researchers, being the producers of epidemiologic data, are in a key position when it comes to choosing pertinent topics, carrying out the studies with skill, and interpreting the results correctly. However, the readers of epidemiologic papers also need insight into epidemiology. They must be able to form their own critical opinion of the validity of the results, and they must be in a position to judge whether the researchers have been correct in their conclusions. There are many different kinds of "consumers" of epidemiologic data, such as administrators, other decision makers, and health professionals of various kinds, the largest category being occupational health physicians. The education of these "consumers" has, therefore, become increasingly important.

This book is mainly intended for the consumers, especially occupational health physicians. It should also be useful as a first introduction to epidemiology for those specializing in occupational health and those considering a career in epidemiologic research. Although its main focus is on occupational medicine, and most of the examples refer to this field, many of the principles of epidemiology apply to other disciplines as well. Therefore, professionals starting a career in public health, occupational hygiene, ergonomics, and other preventive fields could benefit from the book. It could also provide administrators active in setting standards with a better understanding of the underlying scientific data.

Since this book is meant to be at an elementary level, the technical aspects of data analysis have been omitted. Those interested in deepening their epidemiologic knowledge by including data analysis in their field of competence are recommended to consult more advanced textbooks, e.g., Rothman,[4]

Checkoway et al.,[1] and Elwood.[2] Miettinen's[3] outstanding book, *Theoretical Epidemiology,* is suited for very advanced studies; however, the text is best understood if read in conjunction with a training course in epidemiology.

The first chapter of this book gives an introduction to the nature of non-experimental research and points out the ways in which such studies differ from experimental research. The second chapter introduces the most central measures used in epidemiologic research. In the third chapter data sources are presented briefly. The fourth is a presentation of epidemiologic study designs, and the fifth discusses validity problems and generalization. The sixth chapter is a more specific review of problems encountered in epidemiologic studies of five major problem areas, namely, cancer, coronary heart disease, chronic, nonspecific respiratory diseases, musculoskeletal disorders, and psychosocial problems. In chapter seven an outline is given for writing a study protocol, and chapter eight addresses ethical aspects. The last chapter gives an orientation of the interpretation of epidemiologic studies and discusses reasons for false negative and false positive results.

Because epidemiology, being an abstract item, is often difficult to understand for the beginner, I have illustrated the text with numerous examples. I have also tried to simplify many matters, maybe to an extent that would cause senior epidemiologists to raise their eyebrows. However, from my own experience, first as a student and later as a teacher of epidemiology, I have found that the fundamentals are not understood if too many complicated details and conditional statements are served too early in the learning process. This book is, indeed, not written for my learned colleagues. It is intended to be an easily understood introduction to occupational epidemiology for occupational health practitioners.

I believe that many potential readers of this book represent the ''consumers'' of epidemiology. The chapters dealing with basic epidemiologic measures, validity aspects, the epidemiology of some common diseases, and the interpretation of study results are especially written for those people. The fundamentals of study design must also be known to readers of epidemiologic studies to ensure a better understanding. However, some chapters, for example, parts of the chapters on study design and guidelines for a study protocol, are more directed to those starting their research career.

I would like to express my thanks to many of my colleagues who have given constructive criticism to different versions of the manuscript. The comments by Markku Nurminen, Ph.D., D.Sc., and Timo Partanen, M.Sc., have been especially helpful. Georgianna Oja, B.A. checked most of the English language and helped edit the manuscript. Ms. Tarja Hokkanen did much of the typing, and Ms. Ritva Järnström drew the figures. My sincerest thanks are due to all of them.

Professor Olli S. Miettinen has been my teacher in epidemiology. Since 1972 I have had the pleasure of enjoying several of his excellent advanced courses offered annually in Helsinki. Throughout my text is influenced by his thinking. If there are misunderstandings in which the text does not agree precisely with his dogma, the fault is entirely mine.

The Finnish Work Environment Fund has supported this book with a grant that made it possible for me to be on leave from my work at the Institute of Occupational Health, Helsinki, during the summers of 1988, 1989, and 1990. Its support has been crucial for the writing of this book.

REFERENCES

1. Checkoway, H., N. E. Pearce, D. J. Crawford-Brown. *Research Methods in Occupational Epidemiology* (New York: Oxford University Press, 1989).
2. Elwood, J. M. *Causal Relationships in Medicine: A Practical System for Critical Appraisal* (Oxford: Oxford University Press, 1988).
3. Miettinen, O. S. *Theoretical Epidemiology: Principles of Occurrence Research in Medicine* (New York: John Wiley & Sons, 1985).
4. Rothman, K. J. *Modern Epidemiology* (Boston: Little, Brown and Company, 1986).

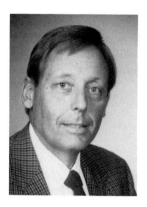

About the Author

Sven Hernberg, M.D., Ph.D. was born in 1934 in Helsinki, Finland. He graduated in medicine from the University of Helsinki in 1959 and became a specialist in occupational medicine in 1964. In 1967 he received his Ph.D. with a thesis on the effects of lead on the red blood cell membrane. In 1960 he joined the National Institute of Occupational Health in Helsinki, first as a research assistant and later as a specialist physician in occupational health. In 1972 he was nominated director of the newly established department of epidemiology and biostatistics and, in 1974, became research director of the Finnish Institute of Occupational Health, an organization which now has a staff of over 500.

Professor Hernberg has been active in many international organizations. He has often been a temporary adviser to the World Health Organization (WHO) and the International Agency for Research on Cancer (IARC). In 1980 he founded and was nominated Chairman of the Scientific Committee on Epidemiology in Occupational Health under the auspices of the International Commission on Occupational Health, the world's oldest international organization in its field, founded in 1906. In 1981 he was elected Vice President of the International Commission and, in 1987, its President, a position he holds until 1993. In 1986 he was elected Honorary Member of the Royal College of Physicians of Ireland as well as of the Royal College of Physicians of London, Faculty of Occupational Medicine. He became a Member Through Distinction of the Canadian Board of Occupational Medicine in 1990. He is a member of several other international organizations.

Professor Hernberg has published over 260 scientific original articles, reviews, and book chapters related to many topics of occupational health, primarily in the areas of clinical occupational toxicology and occupational epidemiology. His main topics have been lead toxicology, solvent toxicology, and occupational cancer. He has been the Editor-in-Chief of the Scandinavian Journal of Work, Environment, and Health since 1974, and is a member of the editorial board of several other international journals.

Table of Contents

CHAPTER 1

Introduction

The first study that could be labeled epidemiologic in the field of occupational medicine was published in 1775 by Sir Percival Pott, who drew attention to the remarkably high occurrence of scrotal cancer among chimney sweeps. Although Sir Percival could not explain the mechanism of the disease, he was able see the connection between an occupational exposure, the sweeping of chimneys, and this type of cancer. The precise etiology of the disease became clear later. Chimney sweeps began working early in old England because only young boys had room to enter the chimneys and do the work from the inside. Their clothing became impregnated with soot, which contains several polycyclic aromatic hydrocarbons and other combustion products, many of them carcinogenic. Especially skinfolds, such as the scrotum, had almost permanent contact with the carcinogenic soot because, in those days, neither the clothing nor the skin was washed frequently.

Sir Percival's observation is an example of how an epidemiologist can infer a causal connection between an exposure and a disease even though the biologic mechanism of action is unknown. There are several other instances where the observation of an epidemiologic association has provided the first clue of a causal connection between an exposure and a disease, long before the mechanism was known. Among the early studies are those of Pirchan and Sikl,[7] who showed that nearly half of the miners in the gold and silver mines in Joachimsthal and Schneeberg died from lung cancer (later shown to be due to radon daughters), of Sir Richard Doll,[3] who demonstrated an excess of lung cancer among gas workers, and of Case and his co-workers,[1] who showed an extremely high excess of bladder cancer among workers exposed to aromatic amines in the production of dyestuffs.

However, in spite of isolated observations like Sir Percival's, it took more than 150 years for epidemiologic methods to become established in the study of work-related diseases. The studies of Doll and Case et al. can be said to represent the beginning of modern occupational epidemiology. The long delay can be partly explained by the underdevelopment of noninfectious disease epidemiology in general; the epidemiologic study of chronic degenerative and neoplastic diseases was not common until the 1950s. Another explanation could be that occupational medicine was mainly a clinical discipline well into the 1960s, and it is still so in some countries. As long as cases of frank clinical occupational disease are common, there is little motivation to study early manifestations or late sequels detectable only at the group level. Besides, the cause of a typical case of occupational disease is evident even without any research at all. Everyone with basic knowledge of occupational medicine realizes that the etiology of lead poisoning is lead exposure.

The last three decades have changed the nature of occupational medicine in the developed world. Frank, classic manifestations of occupational diseases have become less frequent. Some disease forms, for example, lead palsy, manganism, silicotuberculosis, and benzene-induced bone marrow aplasia, have all but disappeared. Subclinical effects, or long-term effects, of occupational exposures are now the main concern. Consequently, the interest of researchers has shifted to the study of such effects. These manifestations are usually nonspecific and they cannot always be linked to a particular exposure or combination of exposures by an individual-centered clinical approach. Establishing a cause-effect relationship between a disease manifestation and an occupational exposure usually requires the study of a group of individuals, sometimes even large populations. Therefore an epidemiologic approach is needed.

A classic occupational disease represents one extreme of a continuum. The other is represented by those work-related diseases whose etiology is occupational to a minor degree only. Even diseases whose etiology is primarily nonoccupational, but whose manifestations become aggravated or exacerbated by occupational factors, can be considered work-related. For example, if a sports injury of the back becomes worse because of a stooped position at work, the symptoms are considered work-related. The World Health Organization (WHO) has recently defined work-related diseases as encompassing the whole of this spectrum, not merely typical, compensable occupational diseases (see also Chapter 6).[4,9] The study of such multicausal morbidity has recently become the other main task of occupational epidemiology.

The identification of single *etiologic factors* of a disease with a multicausal etiology, in this instance the occupational etiologic fraction (see Chapter 4 for a definition), requires refined epidemiologic techniques—the more refined, the smaller the factor of interest. Even small occupational etiologic factors can be important to identify because the cause can usually be removed by preventive action at the workplace.

Work-related diseases characterized by a long, silent latency period between the onset of exposure to the causal factor and the manifestation of disease, are also gaining more importance in occupational medicine. Many chronic degenerative diseases belong to this category, for example, degenerative musculoskeletal disorders, cardiovascular diseases, and many lung disorders. Work-related cancer is probably the most studied of such work-related diseases.

These are some of the challenges that have led occupational medicine to develop from a clinical to a more epidemiologically oriented discipline. In occupational medicine prevention is not only important, it is also much more often possible than in other fields of medicine. In principle (although not always in practice, of course), the prevention of occupational risks is simple. First, the etiologic agent must be identified, next, its effects should be quantified, and then the agent should be removed. Epidemiologic research has a major role in the two first steps of this activity by helping to identify and quantify occupational risks.

PLACE OF EPIDEMIOLOGY IN SCIENCE

Epidemiology has been defined and redefined many times. According to one of the simplest and clearest definitions:

Epidemiology is the discipline of the occurrence of human illness.

Epidemiology has long been viewed as the parent discipline of public health, and it, indeed, has a strong association with preventive medicine. Epidemiologic research is often used in support of health administration and planning, in risk assessment, and in the evaluation of the efficacy of medical treatments. Recently, epidemiologic methods have also been applied to the evaluation of the delivery of health care services. Scientific uses of epidemiology include the study of causes of diseases, the description of their clinical course, the evaluation of the efficacy of medical treatment, and the study of the efficacy of preventive trials. Without, in any way, underestimating the importance of the administrative applications of epidemiologic research, this book focuses mostly on the scientific use of epidemiologic methods, especially their use in the study of causes of disease.

Epidemiology is the discipline of the occurrence of human illness.

The epidemiologic study of work-related diseases can be either descriptive or etiologic (often the term ''analytic'' is used for ''etiologic''). The central issue in occupational epidemiology is to link the occurrence of morbidity to exposures at work (the term ''exposure'' is used throughout this text in a very broad sense), that is, *to study the occurrence of diseases in relation to their work-related determinants*. Hence, occupational epidemiology deals with the *occurrence relation between work-related diseases and the factors determining their outbreak and course*. ''Occurrence relation'' is a term that Miettinen has used particularly for describing the study of the relation of an outcome parameter (morbidity) to its determinants (characteristics on which the morbidity depends).[6] One can say that the study of occurrence relations is the very objective of epidemiologic research.

The occurrence relation can be viewed in both descriptive and causal terms. Finding *causal relations* (to the extent that epidemiologic research can provide the basis for judging the probability of causality, see Chapter 9) is the first step in the investigation of an etiologic problem. One of the most important aspects of occupational medicine is prevention; effective prevention is not feasible without knowing the causes of the disease that should be prevented. The next step is to characterize the occurrence relation in terms of factors modifying it. Description of the quantitative aspects of an occurrence relation is not always needed for understanding the nature of a scientific problem, but this knowledge is important for establishing exposure–effect and exposure–response relationships, which are important for the administrative activity of setting norms and standards (see Chapter 3).

Each disease or injury has its own epidemiology. Hence, terms such as cancer epidemiology, accident epidemiology, and cardiovascular disease epidemiology are commonly used. The term "occupational epidemiology" can be considered an abbreviation of "occupational disease epidemiology"; it would thus fit into a *disease-centered* classification. On the other hand, occupational epidemiology could also be thought of as being *determinant-centered*, in which case it would encompass the study of *all health consequences*, both deleterious and preventive, arising from occupational factors. The fact that neither system of classification covers all that is done in the name of occupational epidemiology can serve as an example of the disarray that still hampers epidemiologic thinking.

The common denominator for the epidemiologic study of various diseases and accidents is *nonexperimental methodology,* which is similar for all such studies in most relevant aspects, although differences in details do exist. Indeed, journals of epidemiology show how diverse is the subject matter of "epidemiology". In the same issue one can find articles on (the epidemiology of) measles, spontaneous abortion, cancer, low-back disease, cardiovascular diseases, acquired immunodeficiency syndrome, occupational accidents, and many other conditions as well. Even disciplines other than medicine, for example, sociology, psychology, and veterinary medicine, even forestry (e.g., in the study of the "epidemiology" of acid rain effects), use nonexperimental research methods of a similar character. The traditional meaning of epidemiology has, however, denoted the study of human illness (Greek: "*epi demos,*" upon the population).

Earlier, infectious diseases were the main targets of epidemiologic research and epidemiology was long considered synonymous with the study of epidemics. Infectious diseases are often acute in the sense that the incubation period between exposure to the infectious agent and the outbreak of the disease is short (numerous exceptions exist, however, such as tuberculosis, leprosy, and human immunodeficiency virus infection). When the incubation period is short, the cause–effect relationship is easy to reveal, and the methodological requirements are less compelling than for chronic diseases with long latency periods. Currently, the emphasis of epidemiologic research is shifting toward the study of noninfectious diseases. Although some of these diseases are acute, most are chronic in the sense that they need a long period of time to develop. The etiology of chronic noninfectious diseases is also more complex than that of most infections. These circumstances place stricter requirements on the epidemiologic methodology used. The interpretation of the results of a study also becomes more difficult.

Epidemiologic research is nonexperimental with the exception of clinical trials and perhaps some other types of intervention studies (see Chapter 4). There are fundamental differences between experimental and nonexperimental research. In *experiments*, the researchers can devise controlled and scientifically optimal conditions. They can decide what individuals (usually experimental animals) will be allocated into the exposed and unexposed categories. In addition, they can decide the exposure conditions (e.g., strength, duration, and degree of variation). They can also ensure that no interfering exposures occur, and can standardize other environmental factors that could interfere with the phenomenon under study (food, light, and temperature, etc.). The outcome variables can also be measured under controlled conditions. By contrast, in nonexperimental research, the researchers have little or no influence on these conditions. This is a severe obstacle in the study of causal connections. Therefore, the experimental approach has many advantages over the nonexperimental one in etiologic studies. The most decisive of these is the possibility to randomize the subjects, which can only be done in experimental research.

Randomization means that the subjects, animals or humans, are randomly allocated into the exposed and unexposed group. The purpose of randomization is to eliminate systematic errors due to properties of the study subjects, such as age, genetic properties, and nutritional state. If the randomization succeeds, these properties will be symmetrically distributed across the groups. The larger the groups, the greater the likelihood for successful randomization. However, if the groups are small, randomization can fail due to chance. It is like tossing a coin 100 or 10 times. In the former instance, the likelihood of an equal distribution between heads and tails is greater than in the latter.

In nonexperimental research, valid study conditions must be created by other methods. If systematic errors cannot be avoided, the results become distorted, and their interpretation difficult, sometimes even impossible. These problems are addressed in Chapter 5.

Although experiments are usually stronger than nonexperimental studies for establishing causal relationships, epidemiology still has an important role in medical research, for many reasons. First, it is most natural to study human disease in man himself. Second, human experiments on harmful exposures are seldom ethically acceptable. Therefore, there are only few problems in occupational medicine that can be studied in human experimentation. Third, many work-related diseases require years or even decades to develop. Experiments of such duration are not feasible. Fourth, there are no good animal models for certain diseases, for example, lumbar disorders, which therefore must be studied in humans themselves. Finally, extrapolation from experimental animals to man is full of problems due to differences in genetic structure, metabolism, behavior, and so on.

Such considerations explain why epidemiologic research has been, and still is, an important source of medical knowledge. Occupational medicine is no exception. Human beings are continuously being exposed to a great variety of biological, chemical, and physical factors in their work environment. Although the goal of occupational medicine is to create healthy work conditions, the fact that such exposures continue cannot be denied. Workplace levels of exposure are, in general, orders of magnitude higher than those occurring in the general environment. Industrial workers can, therefore, serve as a model for the study of the effects of environmental factors, and the opportunity for the extrapolation of toxicologic and other knowledge to the population at large gives occupational medicine, including epidemiology, a wider perspective than the field proper would presuppose—a fact that, unfortunately, is frequently overlooked by researchers and administrators active in the field of public health. It is irrational not to take advantage of the exposure situations the industrialized society has created, even though the conditions are rarely ideal from the scientific point of view.

LEVELS OF EPIDEMIOLOGIC RESEARCH

It has already been stated that epidemiology has an important role in public health administration as a basis for decision-making. On the other hand, epidemiologic research is central for the scientific study of occurrence relations between the manifestations of diseases and their determinants. The methods of research into these two problem areas differ to some extent.

Epidemiologic research is usually classified into three levels: (1) descriptive epidemiology, (2) etiologic (analytic) epidemiology, and (3) interventive (experimental) epidemiology. One may argue whether interventive epidemiology should be on the same hierarchical level as the first two categories. Interventive epidemiology can be viewed as one of the methods by which etiologic problems can be solved. Along these lines of thinking, the classification of interventive epidemiology as a third level could lead to conceptual confusion between study objectives and methodology. However, interventions can also be undertaken to reduce the disease frequency in a population, having practical (public health) goals only.

Descriptive epidemiology is concerned with the occurrence of disease or its manifestations in different populations without any view of causal interpretation of the relation. It may be of interest to know, for example, the connection between age and low-back pain or between the occurrence of headache and work in various departments of a plant, without any ambition of causal interpretation. One may also be interested in the occurrence of hypertension in a workplace only to determine the resources needed for the management of blood pressure control. In the realm of occupational health, descriptive problems may, for example, further concern ''group diagnoses'' of workplaces or occupational groups, the identification of work-related health problems, the monitoring of changes in work conditions, and the determination of normal values for biochemical variables or for concentrations of xenobiotics (foreign chemicals) in the human organism. It is also often said that descriptive epidemiology can generate hypotheses for etiologic research. However, in this instance, the border between ''descriptive'' and ''etiologic'' is not sharp.

Etiologic epidemiology investigates the *causality* of an occurrence relation between diseases and genetic or environmental factors (determinants). The simplest relation is a *crude relation*, which means that factors distorting it or modifying it are not yet identified. A crude relation does not give a full or even correct picture of the occurrence relation. A relation can be modified by a number of factors, for example, immunity or susceptibility, other concomitant disease determinants, and so forth. These *effect modifiers* must also be measured, and their effects assessed in order to give a more complete picture of the nature of the occurrence relation. Furthermore, the occurrence relation can be distorted by extraneous factors—systematic errors such as *confounders* (Chapter 5)—which must be controlled for in the study to reflect the correct nature of the occurrence relation. Both effect modifiers and confounders should be measured and considered in the study of causal relations. It must be stressed that the causality of a relation cannot be directly observed—it must be inferred—and inferences are abstract.

Qualitative epidemiology deals with the very existence of the occurrence relation between two phenomena, the determinant and the disease. It investigates whether a particular exposure *causes* a certain disease. In occupational medicine, qualitative epidemiology investigates the connection between occupational exposures (in a broad sense), on the one hand, and diseases, syndromes, and functional disturbances, on the other. Most diseases have multiple causes, and a central issue is to establish whether work-related factors are among the causes of multicausal diseases.

Quantitative epidemiology investigates the dose–effect and dose–response relationships between exposure and disease when their qualitative connection has already been established, that is, how much disease is caused by different levels and durations of exposure. In occupational medicine this type of research is mostly utilized for establishing a scientific basis for hygienic standards and norms.

Interventive epidemiology, when applied for solving etiologic problems, actively studies the effects on morbidity of changing exposure conditions. Interventive epidemiology bears some resemblance to experimental research (and is, therefore, often called experimental epidemiology), but, as long as randomization cannot be done, it differs fundamentally from true experimental research. (Clinical trials, one of the types of interventive epidemiology, are true experiments.) Interventive epidemiology can be used to study whether an observed association between two phenomena is truly causal. If a change in the exposure changes the morbidity, the likelihood of the causality of a connection becomes more credible. By interventive epidemiologic methods one can also study the efficacy of health care programs. Only few intervention studies have been published in the field of occupational medicine.

CAUSALITY

It is important to realize that even if an association is found between two phenomena, the connection cannot automatically be interpreted as causal. An association can, in addition to being causal, be due to bias or chance, or it can be seeming only. All etiologic research, both experimental and nonexperimental, investigates if *one phenomenon (the disease) is indeed caused by the other (the exposure)*, that is, if the observed association is causal. In medicine, the objective of establishing causality between a disease and its determinants is to learn about the etiology of that disease. There is more rationale in *preventing* the disease by removing its causes when its etiology is known, for example, a hazardous occupational exposure. Otherwise prevention is haphazard, although there are some examples of successful prevention without knowledge of the exact cause. For example, John Snow, or anybody else for that matter, did not know the cholera vibrio when he succeeded in stopping the cholera epidemic in London in 1855.

An observed association can be causal, biased, random or seeming.

Apart from being caused by a systematic error or random events, an association between two phenomena, A and B, can either be causal or it can reflect a statistical association without causality.

If A causes B, A is B's true cause. For example, smoking cigarettes, A, causes lung cancer, B. If smoking is "removed" (meaning that it has never occurred or is terminated), the occurrence of lung cancer decreases. Conversely, increase in the consumption of cigarettes results in a higher occurrence of lung cancer.

Sometimes an exposure, A, causes both a disease, B, and some other phenomenon, C, or some phenomenon, D, devoid of any etiologic effect, may be associated with A. Then the disease, B, is statistically associated with both C and D although neither variable is causal for B. For example, smoking cigarettes, A, may cause yellow fingers, C, and the habit is associated with carrying matches, D. Yellow fingers are indeed statistically associated with lung cancer, and so is carrying matches, but they are not the *cause* of the cancer, although an association can be shown. Washing the fingers with a strong detergent or abandoning the habit of carrying matches does not prevent lung cancer.

Especially in the case of acute diseases, there can occur statistical associations between the disease and, say, biochemical abnormalities of the blood chemistry. It can sometimes be difficult to judge if such abnormalities are causes for, or consequences, of the attack. In other words, does A cause B, or is B a consequence of A?

Distinguishing between causal and noncausal associations is central when making etiologic inferences in research. As already mentioned, the researcher must also make sure that the observed association is not biased, meaning that it cannot be explained by a systematic error (see Chapter 5). There must also be a high probability that it is not due to *chance* either (see Chapters 5 and 9).

Causality is, however, more complicated than that. A cause can lead to an effect over several intermediate steps, in which case one can speak of a "causal chain." The causal chain can be expressed as A→B→C→D→E, where A is the exposure, E the disease and B, C, and D precursors of that disease.

> *Example 1.* Suppose that miners who have been heavily exposed to quartz dust between 1900 and 1920 have an excess mortality from right ventricular heart failure (cor pulmonale). The causal chain contains the following steps: quartz dust, A, causes lung fibrosis, B, which causes restrictive lung function impairment, C, which raises the pressure in the pulmonary artery, D, which causes failure of the right ventricle, E.

Similar causal chains exist for many diseases, although all the intermediate steps may not be known. Certain other diseases may have etiologies that are "causal nets" rather than chains, as Friedman has expressed in his book *Primer of Epidemiology.*[5] Coronary heart disease and back disorders are good examples of diseases with "net" etiology.

The cause–effect relation can take the form of a chain or a net.

The concept of a net-formed causality implies several causes, which together not only cause the disease, but which also interact with each other. *Multicausality* is thus a complicated phenomenon, and there are causes of many different types.

A *sufficient cause* of a disease is so defined that it always results in the outbreak of that disease. Sufficient causes are usually complex and composed of several components; sufficient simple causes are rare. Exposure to the influenza virus alone does not necessarily suffice for the outbreak of influenza, for example, when the exposed person is immune because of a recent infection or a vaccination. Susceptibility is then the other component of the sufficient cause that results in the outbreak of influenza. Exposure to lead alone is a sufficient cause for lead poisoning only if the exposure level is high enough—at lower levels of exposure, the higher than average resistance of some exposed individuals protects them from incurring the poisoning. In toxicology "sufficient'' is thus a relative concept that depends both on the dose and on individual resistance.

A sufficient cause always results in the outbreak of the disease.

On the other hand, exposure to a certain toxic agent, say lead, is always a *necessary cause* for the outbreak of the disease. If there is no exposure, the disease in question cannot break out. In other words, lead poisoning cannot develop in the absence of exposure to lead, whereas exposure to lead does not always result in lead poisoning (if exposure is mild or if the subject has a high resistance). ''Sufficient'' and ''necessary'' are thus entirely different concepts. By removing a necessary cause one can prevent the development of the disease without exerting influence on the other components of a sufficient cause.

A disease cannot break out without a necessary cause.

As already stated, there are only few simple sufficient causes. Even though there is no doubt that cigarette smoking causes lung cancer, only a minority of smokers get the disease. Not all of those exposed to *Mycobacterium tuberculosis* incur the disease tuberculosis. Carbon disulfide exposure causes coronary attacks in only part of the exposed. One single factor—such as exposure to a contagious or toxic agent—is not enough for the outbreak of most diseases. To be sufficient, a cause, as a rule, needs many components, often of different types. These components or parts can be called *contributory causes*, and several contributory causes together comprise a sufficient cause.

Suppose that any one of the following combinations can lead to the outbreak of disease X:

$$A + B + C + D$$
or
$$A + B + E + F$$
or
$$A + C + G + H$$

Each combination is a sufficient cause for X. A, which is a component of all combinations is a necessary (but not sufficient!) cause for the development of X. Supposing that several sufficient causes operate in a population (say, smoking, occupational exposure to polycyclic aromatic hydrocarbons, domestic exposure to radon daughters in respect to lung cancer), the relative share or the *etiologic fraction* of each of them can be computed (see Chapter 4). The etiologic fraction is defined as the fraction of cases whose disease was caused by exposure, or the amount of disease caused by each causal factor.

Interactions between different contributory causes may be additive or multiplicative. Because of complicated interaction patterns and overlapping, the sum of singular contributory causes usually exceeds 100%; in fact, its lower limit is 100% and its upper limit can be any figure in excess of that (e.g., References 2 and 8). For example, a necessary cause for an avalanche is snow; hence 100% of avalanches are caused by snow. However, snow is not a sufficient cause because a steep slope is also needed—another necessary, although not sufficient, cause. Therefore, one can also say that 100% of all avalanches are caused by steep slopes. Moreover, it is well known that snow on steep slopes does not always result in avalanches. In addition, the snow must have particular properties, such as certain crystalline composition, the temperature plays a role, and often a triggering event is needed, such as a loud noise or a skier crossing the slope. The sum of the shares of these contributory causes, together making up the sufficient cause that results in the avalanche, by far exceed 100%. The causal pattern of many diseases is similar.

A certain etiologic factor can have a different force of morbidity depending on the concomitant effects of other factors. Such factors are called effect modifiers, and their action is referred to as effect modifying. For example, smoking modifies the effect of asbestos exposure on the incidence of lung cancer so that it multiplies. Similarly, many dusts and irritant gases cause comparatively more bronchial irritation in smokers than in nonsmokers. As a result of effect modifying, the slope of the exposure–response curve changes.

HYPOTHESES IN EPIDEMIOLOGIC RESEARCH

A hypothesis means a tentative piece of scientific knowledge, an assumption of something's nature. One could think of it as being a part of a theory, which is something "bigger." In epidemiologic research, hypotheses usually relate to cause–effect phenomena, meaning that one assumes that exposure A causes disease B.

A scientific hypothesis must be *testable*, which means that it must have consequences whose correctness or incorrectness can be publicly verified (or falsified). Hypotheses that do not pass the tests must be rejected or alternatively modified and retested. The history of medicine is full of examples of false hypotheses and theories, with deleterious consequences for the patients before the misconceptions finally became scientifically tested, rejected, and buried. Let it suffice to mention only a few, such as the belief (one hesitates to use the word "hypothesis" in this context) in the curative effects of venesection, that inflammatory foci cause a number of rheumatoid, renal, and other diseases, that prolonged bed rest is a benefit for a great many diseases, such as coronary infarction, that a number of medicinal preparations have had any curative effect at all, the hypothesis (perhaps that word can be permitted here) that milk protects against lead poisoning, and so on. Hypotheses usually become rejected or modified as a result of new discoveries or well-designed therapeutic or other trials. Epidemiologic research also has a share in this process.

A scientific hypothesis must be testable.

Etiologic epidemiologic research is often carried out to test hypotheses that postulate that some factor causes a particular disease. In occupational epidemiology, the issue is usually to reveal a causal connection between an occupational exposure and a nonspecific disease. In general, the disease is multifactorial, the work-related factor being only one out of several, which means that it is typically not a sufficient cause. If the work-related factor is a sufficient cause, the causality is so evident—and usually well known—that no epidemiologic research is needed. Unknown occupational diseases caused by new chemicals may be an exception; epidemiologic research can be needed to show the connection for the first time.

It was said that etiologic research is concerned with the testing of a study hypothesis. On the other hand, it also evaluates the study hypothesis in relation to its opposite, the *null hypothesis*. Under the null hypothesis, there is no difference between the study groups in contrast to what the study hypothesis postulates. If the result of the study does not fit the null hypothesis, but rather the study hypothesis, the credibility of the latter increases. By contrast, if the result is in accordance with the null hypothesis, the credibility of the study hypothesis decreases. If the result agrees with both hypotheses, the study is uninformative. If it does not fit any of the hypotheses, it speaks in favor of a second, alternative nonnull hypothesis.[6]

Epidemiologic research can also be performed without a prior hypothesis. One can, for example, explore the factors connected with a certain disease or, alternatively, the different disorders caused by a certain exposure. (The epidemiologic jargon for these types of studies is "fishing expedition.")

The simplest form for a scientific hypothesis is "exposure A causes disease B," for example, exposure to asbestos causes bronchial carcinoma. Hypotheses can also be combined to the form "exposure A causes disease B_1, $B_2, \ldots , B_i$," for example, exposure to asbestos causes bronchial carcinoma, pleural mesothelioma, . . . , and asbestosis. The hypothesis can also be reversed or formulated as "disease B is caused by factors (exposures) A_1, A_2,

. . . , A_i," for example, bronchial carcinoma is caused by cigarette smoking, asbestos, chromates, . . . , and foundry dust. There is a conceptual difference between such formulated hypotheses and purely explorative studies without any prior hypothesis, such as "let us explore the factors associated with disease B." Whether or not a prior hypothesis has been formulated has bearing on the choice of one- or two-sided tests in the statistical analysis, and on the weight given to a particular p-value.

A completely nonspecific constellation can take the form "exposures A_1, A_2, . . . , A_i cause the disease B_1, B_2, . . . , B_i." For example, exposure to lead, arsenic, nickel, copper, zinc, cadmium, and sulfur dioxide in a primary smelter causes bronchial carcinoma, carcinoma of the stomach, prostatic carcinoma, and coronary heart disease. This is no hypothesis-testing constellation, rather one generating hypotheses, and the development of a valid and efficient study constellation can be impossible.

In practice, several hypotheses can be tested in the frame of the same study. For example, a case-referent study (see Chapter 4) can be designed to test a specific hypothesis, according to which exposure to chlorinated hydrocarbons causes liver cancer. Because a complete exposure history can be obtained from the same subjects, other hypotheses can also be tested; for example, does exposure to pesticides also cause liver cancer? One can even use some other cancer type as the reference disease and investigate the effect of some other exposure on that disease, the liver cancer cases then being used as referents. Although everything is carried out as one study, formally the study entity comprises several separate substudies, each with its own hypothesis.

REFERENCES

1. Case, R.A.M., M.E. Hosker, D.B. McDonald, and J.T. Pearson. "Tumours of the urinary bladder in workmen engaged in the manufacture of certain dyestuff intermediates in the British chemical industry, part I. *Br. J. Ind. Med.* 11:75 (1954).
2. Cole, P. and F. Merletti. "Chemical agents and occupational cancer," *Environ. Pathol. Toxicol.* 3:399 (1980).
3. Doll, R. "The causes of death among gas-workers with special reference to cancer of the lung," *Br. J. Ind. Med.* 9:180 (1952).
4. El Batawi, M.A. "Work-related diseases: a new program of the World Health Organization," *Scand. J. Work Environ. Health* 10:341 (1984).
5. Friedman, G. *Primer of Epidemiology* (New York: McGraw-Hill, 1974).
6. Miettinen, O.S. *Theoretical Epidemiology: Principles of Occurrence Research in Medicine* (New York: John Wiley & Sons, 1985).
7. Pirchan, A. and H. Sikl, "Cancer of the lung in the miners of Jachymov (Joachimsthal)," *Am. J. Cancer* 15:681 (1932).
8. Rothman, K.J. *Modern Epidemiology* (Boston, MA: Little, Brown,1986).
9. WHO Expert Committee. "Identification and control of work-related diseases," Report of a WHO Expert Committee. WHO, Geneva, 1985, Tech. Report ser. 714.

CHAPTER 2

Some Basic Epidemiologic Measures

Epidemiologic terminology is unfortunately diversified and imprecise. This situation stems from both conceptual and linguistic inexactness. The aim of this chapter is to define and describe some common epidemiologic measures, especially those relevant to occupational medicine. Many measures have several terms, which may or may not have exactly the same meaning. As a rule only one term is presented for each measure, but, whenever parallel terminology is prevalent, synonyms are also given.

CRUDE RATES

In Chapter 1, epidemiology was defined as the discipline of the occurrence of illness in human populations. Epidemiologists distinguish between two main types of populations. One is *dynamic*. A dynamic population has a turnover of individuals. The population of a city or the employees of a company are good examples. People move into a city or become employed by a company, or they move out from the city or quit their employment; they are born and they die. Such a population has a turnover; it is dynamic. The other type of population is a *cohort*. Its members are defined at a certain point in time, for example, at birth or at the beginning of a study, and they remain in the cohort forever, even after death. Consequently, in a cohort there is no turnover of individuals; it is a fixed population.

Illnesses occur in each type of population. Occurrence can mean the *prevalence* or *existence* of a particular state in a population at some point in time ("having the illness"), or, alternatively, it can mean the *incidence* or *appearance* (or disappearance) of a particular state in a population over a period of time ("getting the disease" or "having become cured"). Both of these measures can either be crude (i.e., related to the whole population) or specific (i.e., related to different segments of it, such as age groups).

Prevalence

As the prevalence measures a disease state in a population — not in individuals — the longer the duration of the disease or condition, the more meaningful it becomes. Acute events such as sudden death cannot be measured at all in the form of prevalence. States are either permanent conditions (e.g., blood groups, invalidity), or chronic diseases, such as silicosis and diabetes. Chronic does not necessarily mean irreversible or incurable, only long-standing. For example, back disorders in a lumber camp may cause 7% of the lumber jacks to be on sick leave during a certain day. Then the prevalence of this disorder is 7% during that day. Although the back may be painful for long periods of time, this disorder usually improves.

Prevalence is usually expressed as the *prevalence rate* (PR), i.e., the proportion of ill persons in a population at some point in time, or

$$PR = \frac{\text{number of diseased persons at time t}}{\text{number of persons in the population}}$$

Because the PR is a proportion, it is dimensionless. Usually it is expressed as the number of cases of the disease per 100,000, 10,000 or 1,000 persons, depending on how common the disease is.

Example 1. A screening for diabetes is launched in a company. Suppose 23 cases are diagnosed among 2473 employees. Suppose also that all the employees attended the screening. The P̂R for diabetes in this company would then be 23/2,473 = 93/10,000 = 0.0093 = 0.93%. This information can be used for the planning of regular checks, but it should be related to such factors as age, gender, and race to give more specific information on the occurrence of the disease.

The prevalence rate quantifies the proportion of individuals with a disease in the population at issue.

Previously, one used to distinguish between point prevalence and period prevalence, say, during 1 year. However, the period prevalence is a rather diffuse concept. It is obtained by adding the cumulative incidence (see the later discussion) during the period in question to the point prevalence at the beginning of that period. Such a formal distinction is meaningless in epidemiologic research because, in practice, few studies can measure anything for a very short point in time (say, a day). Hence "prevalence" usually refers to what is detected during the study period without any distinction being made between what was there at the beginning and what came later. If the condition is stable, there is practically no difference between point and period prevalences; if the duration of the disease is short, the difference grows. A proper study design is then needed to describe the prevalence in a way that is meaningful for the very issue of the study.

The prevalence of a disease must not necessarily be thought of as an all-or-nothing matter. One can, for example, classify the disease into subcategories such as mild, moderate, or severe, say, hypertension, and study the prevalence of these states separately, for example, in relation to noise exposure.

Incidence

When an individual incurs a disease, he or she moves from the healthy to the diseased segment (with regard to a specific disease) of the population, or even out of it if the disease is fatal and the population dynamic. Within the population, this movement of individuals from the state of health to that of manifest disease is described by the *incidence*, which is a measure of the occurrence of new cases of a disease in the population within a period of time.

The incidence can be expressed in two ways. The *incidence rate* (IR), or incidence density (ID), describes the number of new cases of a disease in a population during a time period in relation to the size of the population. Its dimension is time^{-1}.

$$IR = \frac{\text{number of new cases during a period of time}}{\text{number of the population during that period}}$$

The number of the population in the denominator can either be its average number during the follow-up period or its size in the middle of that period. If the population is especially large, such as the population of a whole country or its capital, using its size in the middle of the study period is the most feasible.

Example 2. The workers in a brass foundry were followed for 8 years. During that period, 53 new cases of lead poisoning were diagnosed. There was a continuous turnover of workers during the study, but the foundry expanded and increased the number of employees. Suppose the number of workers was 520 at the beginning of the follow-up and it increased steadily to 680 at the end. The incidence rate is computed in the following way:

New cases: 53
Average size of the population: $(520 + 680)/2 = 600$
Follow-up time: 8 years
$\hat{IR} = 53/600 \times 8$ years $= 0.011$/year

The size of a dynamic population is usually not constant over time, nor does it change steadily as in Example 2. Moreover, a cohort can be so defined that new entries are allowed during a period of time, say, 10 years. The denominator can then be constructed by first computing the time "at risk" for each individual and then summing those individual times. The time at risk for each person begins on the first day of follow-up and is defined as the number of years or months he or she is under observation *and* a candidate for the event. The follow-up ends when the individual incurs his or her first attack of the disease (after which he or she is no longer "at risk") or when the study is terminated. The follow-up periods of all the individuals are then added to form the denominator, or

$$IR = \frac{\text{number of new cases during the period of time}}{\text{sum of the individual person-times at risk}}$$

Usually time is expressed as person-years, but if the follow-up is short, person-months are more suitable.

Whenever the disease can manifest itself after the termination of exposure (e.g., cancer), person-years must be computed irrespective of whether or not the subject has moved out of the exposure, be it job, occupation, geographic area, or something else. By contrast, if the event of interest is sudden and related in time to ongoing exposure (e.g., accident, acute poisoning), it is not meaningful to compute person-years after the subject's exposure has terminated. In the first instance, the population is best studied as a cohort; in the second, the use of a dynamic population is the most convenient.

Sometimes the issue arises of whether several attacks of the disease occurring in the same individual should be counted as incidence. The answer is *"No."* One should always count the first attack only. If the issue is a first attack of lead poisoning as in Example 2, the workers are candidates for incurring poisoning only until they have been poisoned, not in the state of poisoning, or after their cure. However, one could also design a study on the *recurrence* of lead poisoning among those who have had one episode. Then only those who have recovered from their first attack are candidates for recurrence. With the figures from Example 2, the population at risk would be 53, not 600, and person-years should not be computed from the beginning of employment but from the workers' returning to work after the first episode. In both cases, incidence is defined in the same way, namely, as the occurrence among those who can get the event in question, the candidates.[5]

Example 3. Suppose that in the beginning of 1991, we are investigating the occurrence of lung cancer in an iron foundry and that the follow-up started on 1 January 1950 and ended on 31 December 1989. For each single worker the period at risk should then be computed individually. To illustrate how the person-years are computed, let us select 10 employees (A to J) out of a total number of 1000. Let us suppose that the exposure histories of these 10 workers takes the following form:

> A: Began work on 1 January 1950 at 20 years of age.
>   Still working in the foundry.
> B: Began work on 1 January 1950 at 20 years of age.
>   Left employment in 1959.
> C: Began work on 1 January 1950 at 35 years of age.
>   Retired in 1980.
> D: Began work on 1 January 1950 at 20 years of age.
>   Died in 1975.
> E: Began work on 1 January 1960 at 20 years of age.
>   Left employment in 1979.
> F: Began work on 1 January 1953 at 53 years of age.
>   Died in 1967.
> G: Began work on 1 January 1972 at 20 years of age.
>   Still employed.

H: Began work on 1 January 1956 at 20 years of age.
      Worked for two months, quit, and returned in 1961.
      Left employment again in 1966.

I: Began work on 1 January 1951 at the age of 40 years.
      Retired in 1975; died in 1985.

J: Began work on 1 January 1975 at the age of 20 years.
      Still working.

The person-years at risk can now be computed in the following way (no minimum criteria for employment, latency not accounted for, see the later discussion).

Table 1. Computation of Person-Years for Workers A–J in Different Age Categories and Decades of Observation

Age (years)	Decade of Observation				Total
	1950–1959	1960–1969	1970–1979	1980–1989	
20–29	A: 10	E: 10	G: 8	G: 2	65
	B: 10	H: 5	J: 5	J: 5	
	D: 10				
30–39	C: 5	A: 10	E: 10	G: 8	68
		B: 10	H: 6	J: 5	
		D: 10			
		H: 4			
40–49	C: 5	C: 5	A: 10	E: 10	65
	I: 9	I: 1	B: 10	H: 6	
			D: 5		
			H: 4		
50–59	F: 7	C: 5	C: 5	A: 10	51
		I: 9	I: 1	B: 10	
				H: 4	
60–69		F: 8	C: 5	C: 5	28
			I: 9	I: 1	
70–79				C: 5	9
				I: 4	
Total	56	77	78	75	286

The total number of person-years in the subset is 286. Because the disease under study is lung cancer, which takes years to develop, person-years must also be computed after the workers have left the employment (workers B, C, E, H, and J until 1989) but, of course, not after their death (workers D, F, and I). If we now suppose that we had a 1% sample of the cohort, we can say that the real number of person-years was 28,600. If we suppose that the total number of lung cancer cases observed was 15, the $\widehat{IR}$ = 15/28,600 years = 1/1,907 years = approx. 52/100,000 years.

The incidence can also be expressed as the cumulative incidence rate (CIR). This measure is meaningful for fixed populations (i.e., cohorts). The cohort can be an occupational cohort, consisting of workers exposed to a common factor at a certain point in time, or it can be a whole national population, born in a certain year or segments of it. For example, one can study the 50-year incidence of coronary death among men born in 1920 in Manchester, or the study population can be a foundry worker cohort as in Example 4. The CIR expresses the *proportion* of the population that has incurred the disease in question during a certain time period.

$$\text{CIR} = \frac{\text{number of new cases during a time period}}{\text{number of those at risk at the beginning of the period}}$$

The CIR is usually expressed as a percentage, for example, 14% of the Manchester men born in 1920 died of coronary infarction before 50 years of age.

Example 4. Suppose the 30-year lung cancer incidence in a cohort of 2704 foundry workers is studied between 1951 and 1980. Suppose that 78 cases of lung cancer occur. Then,

$$\widehat{\text{CIR}}_{30} = 78/2704 = 0.029 = \text{approx. } 3\%$$

The cumulative incidence rate expresses the proportion of an initially defined population that has experienced the disease at issue during a particular period of time.

The CIR is a function of both the time-specific IR and the length of the follow-up. Even if the time-specific IR remains constant during the follow-up, the CIR increases with time because more individuals get the disease as time passes. Competing causes of death distort the estimate of the CIR, especially when the follow-up time is long, and their effect must be accounted for.

Provided the disease is rare in the study population, and provided both the IR and the mean duration are constant over time, there is a connection between the prevalence, incidence and duration (Figure 1):

$$P = I \times D$$

where P = prevalence
    I = incidence
    D = mean duration

Example 5. Suppose that 120 cases of common cold occur among 750 workers in April, that the incidence is constant, and that the mean duration (sick leave) is 7 days.

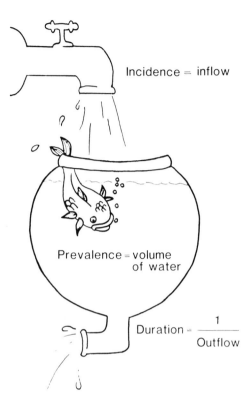

Figure 1. There is a connection between the prevalence, incidence, and duration of a disease.

$$I = (120/750)/\text{month} = 0.16/\text{month}$$
$$D = 7 \text{ days}/30 \text{ days} = 0.23 \text{ months}$$

and

$$P = \frac{0.16 \times 0.23 \text{ months}}{1 \text{ month}} = 0.037$$

In other words, 3.7% of the work force or about 28 workers are, on an average, on sick leave due to common cold each day in April.

If the average duration is not constant, for example, if there are two typical courses of the disease, one without and one with complications, those with the longer duration will be overrepresented among the prevalent cases. Likewise, cancer types with a rapidly fatal course will be underrepresented in a screening program for cancer. This distortion can lead to an incorrect conclusion about the benefits of the screening program. If the benefit is judged merely from comparisons of the survival time of the cases detected in the program, on the one hand, to that of cases found by diagnostic procedures initiated by symptoms, on the other, then an all too optimistic judgment will be made of the efficacy of the screening since the longer duration (from detectability to death) of the cases with a more benign course will result in such cases being overrepresented among the prevalent cases. In such an instance, the prevalent cases are not representative of all cases. By contrast, those patients who seek medical aid because of symptoms have a higher proportion of cancers that would have, in any case, had a more rapid course.

Latency

Many diseases do not become manifest immediately but appear some time after they have been induced. They take time to develop. This time is called the *induction period*. It can be viewed as the time lag from the induction of a chronic disease to its manifestation. However, the exact time of the induction of a chronic disease can only rarely be determined. However, the time of the commencement of the first exposure is usually known. Therefore, the time period between the commencement of exposure and the manifestation of the disease, or the *latency period*, usually serves as a surrogate for the biological induction period in epidemiologic studies even if the onset of exposure does not necessarily result in immediate induction. One can view the latency period as the sum of the preinduction period and the true induction period.

Whenever a chronic disease with a slow course is studied epidemiologically, allowance must be made for the latency period. Hence person-years should not be computed until some time has elapsed from the beginning of exposure. For example, if lung cancer is being studied among asbestos-exposed workers, person-years should not be computed for the first years of exposure. Cases of lung cancer occurring during that period should not be counted either, because the whole period is omitted from the analysis. (Besides, cancers occurring during that period would reflect the background incidence, not the additional risk brought about by asbestos exposure.)

Operationally, the latency period begins immediately after the commencement of exposure and ends when the disease is diagnosed.

Because the latency period is unknown for most diseases, one has to use some approximation in epidemiologic studies. Sometimes it may be possible to estimate a mean latency period from the distribution of the study data, but for most diseases and most exposing agents exact enough data do not exist.

Although most cancers are known to have a long average latency time, its exact length is usually unknown. It has become commonplace to use 20 years as an operational average. Around each average there is a distribution of values, so it would be too strict to disregard the whole period. In cancer epidemiology, half the postulated average, or 10 years, is usually considered the proper time to subtract from the beginning of each person's exposure time. Because it is unlikely that the exposure in question can cause cancers to occur during the first 10 years, the person is not yet "at risk" during these years. Cases occurring during these years are probably due to other causes ("background risk"). There are exceptions, however. Studies of survivors of the Hiroshima bomb have suggested that leukemia has a shorter latency time. Three or maybe five years are therefore a more appropriate approximation for the allowance that should be given the latency time of leukemia in epidemiologic studies. So-called promotors may have an even shorter latency (see Chapter 6). If the latency is poorly known, one could try to allow for two or three different periods and see which one of them gives the most outspoken effect. Whenever the latency period is long, the investigator must design the investigation so that the study population comprises a sufficient number of subjects with a long exposure time (and/or subjects whose exposure took place a long time ago), otherwise the study will be inefficient. If that condition cannot be met, one should seriously consider abandoning the project.

> *Example 6.* Suppose that the issue is to study the lung cancer incidence among insulation workers exposed to asbestos between 1935 and 1990. Worker A was employed in 1940. Supposing that the mean latency time for asbestos-induced lung cancer is 20 years, the computation of person-years starts from 1950, because half the assumed average latency period is 10 years. In 1990 he has accrued 40 person-years (instead of 50). Worker B was employed in 1981. He has been followed for 9 years, but since half the assumed latency time was set at 10 years, he does not belong to the population at risk.

Risk

Incidence and prevalence are group measures (i.e., characteristics of populations, not of single individuals). *Risk* denotes the probability for each single individual to incur the disease in question within a certain period of time (e.g., 1 year, 10 years, a lifetime). Whenever the CIR of a disease is known, it is possible to compute the individual average risk for the members of that population. However, because the risk is a probability, it can never be observed.

> *Example 7.* Suppose that the mortality from coronary heart disease for men aged 51-60 years is 10% in a certain population during a certain time period. Then the average risk for each man belonging to that population is also 10%. However, individuals either die or stay alive, so at the end of the period the

concept is meaningless for the survivors in spite of the fact that the mortality has been 10% for the population. Moreover, such an average risk measure is crude because many factors modify individual risk. By measuring these factors (e.g., blood pressure, serum cholesterol, smoking), one can give a more precise risk estimate, provided a risk function based on that study and containing the relevant factors is available.

Risk is the probability for an individual to incur a certain disease.

Rate Ratio and Rate Difference

The PR and IR describe how common a certain disease is in a population. They are entirely descriptive measures. In order to become scientifically meaningful, they must be compared to some reference value. The PR, ID, and the CIR can be compared by dividing the measure of the exposed group by that of a reference group (see also Chapter 4). Consequently, the ratio of these rates, the *rate ratio* (RR), is the rate of the exposed group (R_{exp}) divided by the rate of the reference group (R_{ref}) or

$$RR = R_{exp}/R_{ref}$$

Common synonyms for the rate ratio are "risk ratio" and especially "relative risk." For reasons stated earlier, "rate" is more correct than "risk" for a population measure.

Example 8. Suppose the issue is to study the coronary mortality of male workers exposed to carbon disulfide. Both the exposed and the reference group comprise 343 men at the start of the study. Let us assume that after 8 years of follow-up, 20 exposed men and 9 referents have died of coronary heart disease, i.e.,

$$\widehat{CIR}_8 \text{ for the exposed} = 20/343 = 0.058 = 5.8\%$$
$$\widehat{CIR}_8 \text{ for the referents} = 9/343 = 0.026 = 2.6\%$$
$$\widehat{RR} = 0.058/0.026 = 2.22$$

The rate ratio is the rate of the exposed group divided by that of the reference group.

If the RR is over 1, the morbidity of the exposed group is higher than that of the reference group and the individual risk to incur the disease is consequently greater for each exposed person than for each referent. If the RR is less than 1, there is less morbidity in the exposed group and the risk of each exposed individual is lower. Provided the study is valid and large enough (see Chapter 5), one can postulate that the exposure in question *causes* the disease in the former case and *prevents* it in the latter.

RR is a *point estimate* ("best guess") and therefore, varies, randomly. Should the same study be repeated, the point estimate of the RR would probably be different due to this random variation. In order to get an idea of the limits within which the variation occurs, one can compute a *confidence interval*, CI, for the RR. A CI is the range which covers the true value of the RR with a certain probability. Usually the CI is expressed as the 95%, sometimes as the 99% interval. However, if the hypothesis tested is unidirectional (the exposure can only cause, never prevent the disease), the 90% interval is preferred (see Chapter 5). If the lower confidence limit is over 1, the $\widehat{RR}$ is statistically significant at the confidence level chosen.

The confidence interval gives limits for the range of random variation of the rate ratio.

The CI_{95} for the CIR is computed from the following formula (N = number of persons):

$$CIR \pm 1.96 \Big/ \sqrt{\frac{CIR\,(1-CIR)}{N}}$$

The CI_{95} for the ID is (T = number of person years):

$$ID \pm 1.96 \Big/ \sqrt{\frac{ID}{T}}$$

The CI_{95} for the RR is:

$$RR^{(1 \pm 1.96/\chi)}$$

where chi is the square root of the χ^2 value used in the significance testing.

Example 9. In Example 8, a CIR of 5.8% was computed for coronary heart disease among workers exposed to carbon disulfide. The CI_{95} is computed in the following way:

$$0.058 \pm 1.96 \,[0.058\,(1-0.058)/343]^{1/2}$$
$$= 0.058 \pm 0.025 = 0.033,\ 0.083 = 3.3\%,\ 8.3\%$$

The statistical significance measure for the difference between the exposed and the unexposed groups is $\chi^2 = 4.35$; hence the CI_{95} for the $\widehat{RR}$ is computed as follows:

$$2.22^{(1 \pm 1.96/\sqrt{4.35})} = 1.04, 4.7$$

Since the lower limit is over 1, the mortality from coronary heart disease among the exposed is statistically significantly elevated.

The absolute difference between two measures of morbidity, the *rate difference* (RD), sometimes also called risk difference or attributable risk, is obtained by subtracting the rate of the reference group from that of the exposed group or

$$CI_{95} = RD = R_{exp} - R_{ref}$$

The CI for the RD is computed as follows:

$$CI_{95} = RD(1 \pm 1.96/\chi)$$

Example 10. With the numbers from Example 8, the $\widehat{RD} = 0.058 - 0.026 = 0.032$. In other words, for each 1000 exposed men, the 8-year excess mortality from coronary heart disease is 32 (CI_{95} 22 to 58) cases.

The rate difference is computed by subtracting the rate of the reference group from that of the exposed group.

Odds Ratio

So far measures typical of cohort and cross-sectional studies (see Chapter 4) have been presented. In case-referent studies direct estimates of the PR or IR cannot be obtained. Instead, the comparison concerns differences in exposure frequencies between cases and referents. Thereby an *indirect* estimate of the RR can be computed. The structure of the case-referent design is presented in Chapter 4. In short, patients having the disease under study, the cases, are gathered from the study base. A sample of persons without that disease are drawn as referents. Next their exposure histories are gathered, either with regard to a specific exposure, say, chlorinated hydrocarbon solvents, or with regard to all relevant exposures, for example, the entire occupational history. Then the exposures are classified and coded, and the cases and referents are classified as "exposed" and "nonexposed" with regard to one exposure at a time. Minimum criteria for "exposure" must be preset.

The number of exposed cases is then divided by that of the unexposed ones, and the number of exposed referents by that of the unexposed referents. The result is the ''odds'' for having been exposed if one is either a case or a referent. From these ''odds'' the *odds ratio* (OR) is computed as follows:

$$OR = \frac{\text{exposed cases/unexposed cases}}{\text{exposed referents/unexposed referents}}$$

The OR, the RR, and the RD are all discussed further in Chapter 4.

STANDARDIZED MEASURES OF MORBIDITY

The morbidity of a population depends on its specific properties, especially its distributions of age, gender, social group, and race. It may also depend on the calendar time of the study. Age is an important determinant of morbidity, especially for chronic degenerative diseases and neoplastic diseases. Men and women have different morbidity rates from many diseases, such as coronary heart disease, several types of cancer, and peptic ulcer. For certain other diseases, for example, most infections, there are no such differences. Morbidity is usually higher in the lower social categories. In multiracial countries, such as the United States, race is also a relevant determinant of morbidity. In American epidemiologic studies it is a rule to separate ''whites'' and ''non-whites.'' The differences in morbidity found between different ethnic groups, is to a great extent, explained by social factors. Also religion may be important; for example, alcohol-related diseases are rare among Muslims. Many diseases have become more or less frequent during the last 50 years or so. For example, in developed countries tuberculosis has decreased, whereas lung cancer has increased, first among men and later among women. Coronary heart disease increased until the 1970s, when it reached a plateau, and then started to decrease in the 1980s in many industrialized countries.

Such characteristics of populations must always be considered when their morbidity rates are being compared. Crude measures describe the population without allowing for these properties. As already has been shown, a crude rate is simply computed so that the number of cases is divided by the number of persons or person-years in the population. Crude rate ratios and rate differences are computed according to the same principle. However, crude measures for two or more populations can be compared only if the populations have similar relevant properties. Usually this is not the case. Therefore the crude measures must be adjusted or standardized to make the comparison meaningful.

Adjustment means that some distribution, say, the age distributions of the study and the reference population are artificially changed so that they correspond to a common standard age distribution. For example, if someone is interested in the mortality of the study population, that person must first make sure that its age structure corresponds to that of the reference population. If this is not so, which is usually the case, it must be adjusted. This adjustment is called age standardization, which means that the age distributions of both populations are adjusted to a common age distribution. The common distribution can be that of the study population, that of the reference population, or their combined age distribution. Any population can, in principle, be used as the standard, and many populations can be standardized to the same standard population.

In occupational epidemiology, the age distribution of the exposed population is often preferred as the standard because the phenomenon of interest occurs in that population.[8] Adjustment can also be done for a number of other factors, for example, for the sake of controlling confounding by various factors (see Chapter 5).

Standardization is one of the methods of adjustment; it can be direct or indirect. Example 11 concerns *direct standardization* of a mortality rate. The standardization is done for age, and the age distribution of the exposed population is taken as the standard. The incidences of the reference population in each subcategory are, therefore, given weights corresponding to the distribution in the exposed population. The observed numbers of "cases" in each age category of the reference population are thereby changed to what they would have been, had the referents' age distribution been that of the exposed population. The rates can now be directly compared within each age category and for the whole populations to yield the *standardized rate ratio* (SRR).

Example 11. Suppose the mortality of two populations with different age structure should be compared. The properties of these tentative populations are shown in Table 2.

Table 2. Mortality of Two Hypothetical Populations, For Example, During 5 Years

Age (years)	Number of Population		Number of Deaths		Mortality rate per 1,000	
	Exposed	Reference	Exposed	Reference	Exposed	Reference
30–39	3000	1000	15	5	5	5
40–49	2000	2000	20	10	10	5
50 +	1000	3000	20	39	20	13
Total population	6000	6000	55	54	9.2	9.0

For the sake of simplicity, both populations have been given the same size, and the total number of deaths is almost the same. The crude mortality rates are 9.2 and 9.0 per 1000, respectively. Because the age structure of the populations is different—the reference population being older—these crude rates are not comparable. For achieving comparability, the age structure of the reference population is now artificially adjusted so that it is similar to that of the exposed population (direct standardization, see below), the exposed population being used as the "standard." This adjustment is made by calculating the number of deaths that *would have occurred* in the reference population if it had had the same age distribution as the exposed population and the same age-specific mortality rates that were observed.

Exposed: (0.005 × 3000) + (0.010 × 2000)
(0.020 × 1000) = 55

These numbers are the real ones because the exposed population has been used as the standard.

Reference: (0.005 × 3000) + (0.005 × 2000)
(0.013 × 1000) = 38

Here the *rates* are real, but the *number* of persons in each age group has been artificially adjusted to correspond to the distribution in the exposed population.

The directly standardized mortality rates can now be computed as follows:

Exposed: (55/6000) × 1000 = 9.2%
(exactly as in Table 2)
Reference: (38/6000) × 1000 = 6.3%
(using the standardized rate)
SRR = 9.2/6.3 = 1.46

Example 11 was a simplified exercise of direct standardization; the numbers in Example 12 have been taken from a published study (M. Numinen, personal communication).[7]

Example 12. The mortality of physicians from cardiovascular diseases was compared with that of some other well-educated occupational groups. Table 3 shows how the observed cases of death were directly standardized. The age distribution of the physicians was used for weighing the distributions of the other groups.

Table 3. Mortality from Cardiovascular Diseases among Physicians Compared with that of Managers and Lawyers

Age group	Physicians			Managers		Lawyers	
	Person years	Weight	Deaths	Person years	Deaths	Person years	Deaths
30–34	1,671	0.0724	—	2,471	1	786	—
35–39	4,799	0.2079	1	8,755	5	2,225	—
40–44	5,466	0.2368	7	14,493	15	2,717	1
45–49	3,607	0.1563	5	16,934	37	2,878	7
50–54	2,559	0.1109	7	15,818	72	2,970	16
55–59	2,101	0.0910	15	12,806	81	2,667	19
60–64	1,666	0.0722	31	10,150	118	2,490	29
65–69	1,016	0.0440	17	5,124	84	1,371	23
70–74	195	0.0084	4	939	21	252	9
Total	23,080	1.0	87	87,490	434	18,356	104

The crude mortality rate for the physicians per 1000 person-years was 87 × 1,000/23,080 = 3.77. The corresponding figure for managers was 434 × 1,000/87,490 = 4.96, and for lawyers 104 × 1,000/18,356 = 5.67.

The standardized mortality rate for the managers was computed from each age category by using the proportion of physicians in each age category as weights, as follows:

$$0.0724 \times (1/2471) + 0.2079 \times (5/8755) + \ldots +$$
$$0.0085 \times (21/939) = 0.00356 = 3.56/1000 \text{ person-years}$$

The SRR for the lawyers was computed in the same way. The results showed that the mortality rates were rather similar in all the occupational groups even if the crude rates differed considerably.

Table 4. Crude and Standardized Mortality Rates and Standardized Rate Ratios (SRR) for Managers and Lawyers Compared with Those of Physicians

	Physicians	Managers	Lawyers
Crude mortality/ 1000 person years	3.77	4.96	5.67
Age-standardized mortality/ 1000 person years	(3.77)	3.56	3.60
SRR (comparison with physicians)	(1.00)	0.94	0.96

Whereas direct standardization uses weights proportional to the age-specific sizes of the "standard" population, *indirect standardization* is a process in which the standard supplies a set of rates instead of the weighting distribution. This set is weighted to the age distribution of the population of interest, the "exposed" population. Indirect standardization generates an "expected" rate or an expected number for the crude rate or the number of cases observed in the study population.

Standardization is the adjustment of two or more rates to a common distribution.

Example 13. Suppose the mortality of an exposed population should be compared with that of the general population by indirect standardization. Suppose also that both the number of observed deaths and the mortality of the general population are as shown in Table 5.

Table 5. Indirect Standardization

Age (years)	Exposed Population			General Population		
	Person years	Cases	Crude Rate × 10^{-5}	Person years	Cases	Crude Rate × 10^{-5}
35–54	4,711	3	63.7	2,457,600	1,800	73
55–64	28,585	77	269	924,500	2,200	238
35–64	33,296	80	240	3,382,100	4,000	118

The crude rate ratio is 240/118 = 2, but because the exposed group is older than the reference population, age confounds the comparison (see Chapter 5). By indirect standardization, one compares the number of cases observed in the exposed group with those that *would have occurred* in it, had it had the same age-specific rates as the reference population.

$$35 \text{ to } 54 \text{ years:} \quad 4{,}711 \times 73.3 \times 10^{-5} = \quad 3.45$$
$$55 \text{ to } 64 \text{ years:} \quad 28{,}585 \times 238 \times 10^{-5} = \quad 68.03$$

The sum of these expected numbers is 71.48. The age-standardized $\widehat{RR}$ is 80/71.48 = 1.12. and hence there is very little difference between the mortality of the populations.

The most widely used and best known indirectly standardized ratio is the *standardized mortality ratio* (SMR). Traditionally this ratio is used when the mortality of an exposed group is being compared with that of the general population. It is computed as follows:

$$SMR = O/E \times 100$$

where

O = number of observed cases in the exposed group
E = number of cases expected in the exposed population,
    given the mortality (morbidity) of the reference population

The ratio O/E is usually multiplied by 100, and therefore the SMR is 100 times the RR. If the SMR is higher than 100, the mortality is increased among the exposed. An SMR lower than 100 is more difficult to interpret whenever the general population has been used as the reference, because a number of extraneous factors usually lower the observed mortality rate among employed workers. This so-called healthy worker effect is discussed in Chapter 5.

The standardized mortality ratio is an indirectly standardized ratio describing the mortality of an exposed population in relation to that of the general population.

Other measures of morbidity can also be compared in the same way provided the expected numbers are available. The abbreviation SMR is sometimes also used for the *standardized morbidity ratio*, when other measures of morbidity are being compared. The term *standardized incidence ratio* (SIR) is preferable; this can be used both for directly and indirectly standardized ratios.

The SMR can be computed either for total mortality or separately for different causes of death (cause-specific mortality). Generally speaking, the total mortality is too crude and nonspecific a measure to give meaningful information about the effects of most exposures, whereas a cause-specific SMR conveys more information. Sometimes a cause-specific SMR is markedly elevated although the SMR for all causes is less than 100.

As already shown in Example 13, the expected numbers are computed from the real rates of the reference population (e.g., national death statistics), but they are adjusted so as to correspond to the age distribution of the exposed population. Example 14 illustrates the computation of the SMR.

Example 14. Koskela et al.[2] studied the mortality of a cohort of foundry workers. They compared the mortality of the foundry workers with that of the general Finnish male population in 1967, that year being representative of the follow-up period. The age-standardized mortality figures for men can be found from the World Health Organization's publication *World Health Statistics Annual.* Table 6 shows how the SMR for all causes was computed.

Table 6. Total Mortality for Foundry Workers

Age (years)	Person Years	Observed Deaths	Deaths in the Population $\times\ 10^{-5}$	Expected Deaths^{-5}	SMR
15–24	8,737	3	114.7	10.0	30
25–34	16,778	29	184.8	31.0	94
35–44	12,866	59	446.4	57.5	103
45–54	6,233	69	1,131.3	70.5	98
55–64	2,184	39	2,642.1	57.7	68
65–74	345	23	5,870.8	20.3	113
75–	17	2	14,615.8	2.5	80
Total	47,160	224	25,005.9	249.5	90

For example, the expected deaths are computed for the age group 15 to 24 years as follows:

$$114.7 \times 8737/10^5 = 10.0$$

The $\widehat{SMR}$ for this category is $3/10 = 0.3 = 30$ and that for the entire cohort is $224/249.5 = 0.898 = 90$.

Because the SMR is computed specifically for each exposed group with the group's own age distribution being used as the standard, it is not correct to compare SMR values of different populations directly. They are not mutually standardized, and the expected values of each population depend on its age structure.[3,8,10] For example, if the SMR for lung cancer of an American cohort of foundry workers is 154 and that of a British cohort is 177, one cannot conclude from these figures alone that the risk of contracting lung cancer is higher among British foundry workers.

Two or more standardized mortality ratios cannot be directly compared because they are not mutually standardized.

PROPORTIONATE MORTALITY

Sometimes the records of an exposed population are so deficient that person-years cannot be computed. Then, the SMR or any other absolute measure of morbidity cannot be computed either, because no denominator is available. If this is so, the total mortality rate cannot be estimated at all and absolute rates for the cause-specific mortality also cannot be computed. However, provided death certificates are available, it is possible to study the cause-specific mortality in *relative terms* by comparing the proportion of deaths due to a specific cause in the exposed group to that of the reference population. This is how the *proportionate mortality ratio* (PMR) is derived. Usually the general population is used as the reference population. Data on the general population can be obtained from national (or regional) death statistics. The PMR should be standardized for age and calendar period. It is computed in the following way:

$$\text{PMR} = \frac{a/(a+c)}{b/(b+d)}$$

where a = number of deaths from the cause under
       study among the exposed
      b = number of deaths from the cause under
       study in the reference population
      c = number of deaths from the remaining causes
       among the exposed
      d = number of deaths from the remaining
       causes in the reference population

Example 15. Suppose we are interested in the mortality of workers employed by a large chemical plant. Suppose that the employer's records are too incomplete to allow computations of person-years. For example, the number of workers employed in the study period 1941 to 1980 is not exactly known, and neither is the time when employment started. However, it is known that altogether 790 male workers died in the period 1951 to 1980, and copies of their death certificates are available. According to the certificates, 174 had died of cancer. Of them, 66 died of lung cancer. For all cancers, a = 174 and c = 616. Then a/(a+c) = 174/790 = 0.22. The corresponding figures for b and d are derived from national (regional) mortality figures, which must be age-standardized to correspond to the age distribution of the deaths in the exposed population. Because the study period spans 30 years, one representative year is not sufficient. Instead, for example, three representative years, say 1955, 1965 and 1975, are selected and the average of these years is used for reference. Let us suppose that $b/(b+d) = 0.18$. Then $\widehat{PMR} = 0.22/0.18 = 1.22$ (i.e., there is a relative overmortality from cancer). The $\widehat{PMR}$ for lung cancer is derived in the same way. Now $a = 66$, $c = 724$, and $a/(a+c) = 0.09$. If $b/(b+d) = 0.06$, then $\widehat{PMR} = 0.09/0.06 = 1.5$. The proportional mortality from lung cancer is rather high, but, since we do not know if the mortality from other causes has been lower than expected in absolute terms, the interpretation must be made with caution.

Although the PMR is simple to compute and it is sometimes the only alternative, one must realize its weaknesses. First, even if the total mortality of the study population is increased, the *proportion* of deaths due to a single disease may not be elevated. True, the absolute rate of that disease may be higher than in the reference population, but, because the total mortality is also elevated, the *proportion* does not necessarily change. Second, the proportionate mortality of the disease under study is influenced by changes in the mortality of other causes. If the share of ''c'' increases, that of ''a'' decreases, irrespective of whether or not the exposure under study had any influence on ''a.'' In other words, if one cause of death is overrepresented, then some others must be underrepresented. The more common the ''other cause,'' the greater the effect. For example, if the exposure in question increases the mortality of both heart diseases and lung cancer (as, e.g., cigarette smoking), it may well be that the increase of deaths from heart diseases, being a common cause of death, masks that of lung cancer in a comparison based on proportionate mortality.

In spite of these considerations, a proportionate mortality analysis can sometimes suggest that a work-related factor increases the occurrence of a specific disease.

Example 16. At the first stage of a study on the effects of carbon disulfide exposure on the occurrence of coronary heart disease, we analyzed the proportionate mortality.[1] We found that 52% of the deaths among those who had been employed by a viscose rayon plant in 1945 to 1966 were due to coronary heart disease. The age-standardized expected value was only 32%. The $\widehat{PMR}$ was thus $52/32 \times 100 = 163\%$, which was statistically significant. A later prospective follow-up showed that, during the first 5 years, 1967 to 1972, 14 deaths from coronary heart disease occurred among the exposed compared to 3 only in a carefully selected reference group. The rate ratio was 4.7, which was statistically significant.[11] This study is discussed in more detail in the examples presented in Chapters 4 and 5.

However, in the absence of data allowing the computation of expected numbers, there is an alternative to the PMR. Instead of taking the ratio of proportions, one can compute the ratio of the odds for the disease of interest.[4] If the same symbols as for the PMR are used, the odds for the exposed are a/c and those for the reference population are b/d. Thus the mortality odds ratio (MOR), is:

$$MOR = \frac{a/c}{b/d}$$

If, instead of using all causes other than the disease in question, one selects a *specific cause* as the reference disease, one that is neither caused nor prevented by the exposure of interest, many of the uncertainties involved in using all other causes as the reference are removed. For example, the MOR is independent of the size of the pool of other causes, especially if the reference cause of death is chosen with insight into the problem.

The formula MOR = (a/c)/(b/d) can also be expressed as ad/bc, which equals the rate ratio (see Chapter 4). In fact, using the MOR instead of the PMR adopts the viewpoint of a case-referent study in which a and b are cases and c and d are referents (as is discussed in more detail in Chapter 4).

EXPOSURE–EFFECT AND EXPOSURE-RESPONSE RELATIONSHIPS

When the qualitative relationship between two phenomena, the exposure and the morbidity, has been established, the next step is to investigate their *quantitative* relationship (i.e., how much disease is caused by different levels of exposure). This information is of fundamental importance in the setting of hygienic standards.

In the realm of pharmacology, the quantitative relationship is based on knowledge of the *dose*. However, in the realm of occupational health, the dose is usually not known, and therefore the concept of *exposure* is more adequate than that of dose. Although *effect* and *response* are often used as synonyms in epidemiology, they have different meanings in pharmacology and toxicology, and a distinction is therefore motivated, at least in occupational epidemiology.

In its meeting in Tokyo in 1974, the working group on toxicology of metals defined *effect* as "the biological change caused by an exposure."[6] When the numerical values for both the exposure and the effect are known, the *exposure–effect* relationship can be computed. The relationship between the concentration of lead in the blood, on the one hand, and the concentration of δ-aminolevulinic acid (ALA) in urine, on the other, may serve as an example. From this relation it is possible to estimate how high the average excretion of ALA in urine is at any average blood lead level. The same working group also defined *response* as the proportion of a population having values showing an abnormal effect (e.g., an ALA concentration exceeding 5 mg/L of urine).

The higher the exposure level, the higher the proportion of individuals having abnormal values. This relationship in called the *exposure–response relationship*.

The exposure-effect relationship thus describes the *average* effect of each exposure level. Since no population is homogeneous, that picture can easily be misleading. The exposure-response relationship shows individual variations in sensitivity better because it describes the *proportion* of the population showing abnormal reactions to each exposure level. Describing the connection between exposure and morbidity in terms of an exposure-response relationship requires "abnormal" to be defined. In the case of an all-or-nothing response, such as cancer, or any death for that matter, this is no problem, but for continuous variables, for example, serum cholesterol level or urinary excretion of ALA, there must be some cut-off point. Argumentation on what is normal and what is not is irrelevant in this context; what matters is that some cut-off point must be defined somewhere within the disputed range.

Example 17. Seppäläinen et al.[9] studied the long-term effects of lead exposure on the conduction velocities of peripheral nerves. The exposure was assessed from earlier measurements of the concentration of lead in the blood (B–Pb). Such measurements were available for the entire exposure period. Three different B–Pb measures were tried (i.e., the time-weighted average B–Pb, the most recent B–Pb and the highest B–Pb ever measured). Of these, the last one correlated best with the nerve conduction velocities and was therefore chosen. The correlation was statistically significant for several nerves; high B–Pb values corresponded to low conduction velocities. Figure 2 illustrates this exposure–effect relationship. The sensory conduction velocity (SCV) of the radial nerve is chosen as an example. The straight line shows the *average* relationship between B–Pb and the SCV. The scatter is large, however, and therefore the information conveyed by the average is restricted.

In this study the exposure–response relationship was also examined. A positive response was defined as a velocity below two standard deviations of the average of a large normal material, previously collected by the Institute of Occupational Health in Helsinki.

Table 7 shows how those with at least one "abnormal" finding were distributed according to exposure category. This method of scrutinizing the relationship shows the proportion of individuals with abnormal values.

Table 7. Example of an Exposure–Response Relationship

Maximal B–Pb (μg/100 mL)	Number	Abnormal values (%)	p
Referents[a]	34	3	
–40	3	..	ns
40–49	11	27	ns
50–59	28	32	0.0046
60–69	19	42	0.0012
70–	17	53	0.00013

[a]The mean B–Pb of the referents was 11 μg/100 mL.

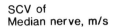

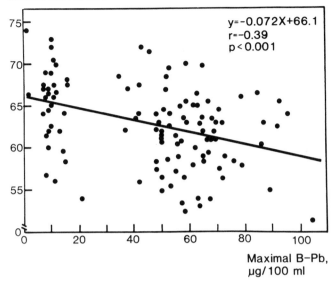

Figure 2. Example of an exposure–effect relationship. The conduction velocity of the sensory impulses in the radial nerve (SCV) are shown in relation to the highest blood lead (B–Pb) value measured during the follow-up period. The measurements were performed on 78 lead workers and 34 referents.

Quantitative epidemiology has both scientific and practical use. Knowledge of the exposure-effect and exposure-response relationships adds to the understanding of a scientific problem. This knowledge is also fundamental for the setting of hygienic norms and standards.

Standard-setting has two steps. The first involves evaluation of existing scientific biomedical knowledge in quantitative terms. On the basis of this evaluation, a safe level of exposure can be defined. "Safe" has many definitions. One is that no adverse effects should be detected at the level defined as "safe." The "safe" level can then be used as the *health-based* exposure limit.

An *administrative standard* is not only a scientific, but also a technological, economic, and societal decision. It is an administrative compromise, different in different countries, while the health-based standard applies more universally, being biological only. In administrative standard-setting, a certain level of risk may be accepted (or rather tolerated). In such situations, the decision becomes fundamentally different from the scientific procedure of defining a health-based standard. The scientist should, of course, also participate in the societal procedure, but only as an adviser, not as a decision-maker.

REFERENCES

1. Hernberg, S, T. Partanen, C.-H. Nordman and P. Sumari. "Coronary heart disease among workers exposed to carbon disulphide," *Br. J. Ind. Med.* 27:313 (1970).
2. Koskela, R-S, S. Hernberg, R. Kärävä, E. Järvinen and M. Nurminen. "A mortality study of foundry workers," *Scand. J. Work Environ. Health* 2 (Suppl. 1):73 (1976).
3. Miettinen, O.S. "Standardization of risk ratios," *Am. J. Epidemiol.*, 96:383 (1973).
4. Miettinen O.S. and J. D. Wang. "An alternative to the proportionate mortality ratio," *Am. J. Epidemiol.*, 114:144 (1981).
5. Miettinen, O.S. *Theoretical epidemiology. Principles of Occurrence Research in Medicine.* (New York: John Wiley & Sons, 1985).
6. Nordberg, G.F. Ed. "Effects and dose-response relationship of toxic metals," in *Proceedings from an International Meeting on the Toxicology of Metals, Tokyo 1974* (Amsterdam: Elsevier, 1976).
7. Rimpelä, A., M. Nurminen, P. Pulkkinen, M. Rimpelä, and T. Valkonen. "Lääkärien kuolleisuus: auttaako ammattitaito omassa terveydenhuollossa (Mortality of physicians: does medical skill help in one's own health care?)" *Suom. Lääkäril* 6:474. (1987), (Engl. summary).
8. Rothman, K. J., *Modern Epidemiology* (Boston, MA: Little, Brown 1986), p. 358.
9. Seppäläinen, A.M., S. Hernberg and B. Kock. "Relationship between blood levels and nerve conduction velocities," *NeuroToxicology* 1:313-32 (1979).
10. Silcock, H. "The comparison of occupational mortality rates," *Popul. Stud. (London)* 13:183 (1959).
11. Tolonen M., S. Hernberg, M. Nurminen, and K. Tiitola. "A follow-up study of coronary heart disease in viscose rayon workers exposed to carbon disulphide," *Br. J. Ind. Med.* 32:1 (1975).

CHAPTER 3

Sources of Information

Several countries, especially the Nordic countries Denmark, Finland, Iceland, Norway and Sweden, have good national, and also regional or local, registers, the use of which greatly facilitates epidemiologic research. Many other countries are not in this position. When good registers are lacking, the data must be gathered in other, more cumbersome ways. Unfortunately, in many countries, the increasing public concern for confidentiality has led to legislation restricting the use of registers, sometimes even making it impossible.

In broad terms, registers can be classified into vital statistics, population registers, and exposure registers. Epidemiologic research usually requires the use of several different registers, or alternatively, of other sources of information (Figure 1).

Because both the availability of registers, their type, their quality, and the legislation concerning their use vary significantly from one country to another, it is not possible in this context to describe in detail how registers are kept and how they are used in epidemiologic research. Instead, the focus is more on their general features, which apply irrespective of national conditions. For specific information, researchers should always familiarize themselves with the sources of information in their own country.

VITAL STATISTICS

Death Registers

Death registration is more or less complete in the United States, Canada, Europe, Japan, Australia, and some other industrialized countries, but elsewhere it is deficient. In general, death registers are central, national registers, but there are also state and even local registers, for example, parish registers. The data in the death registers are taken from the death certificates, which usually list the name, the dates of birth and death, the gender and the occupation of the decendent, as well as the primary and contributing causes of death. From the epidemiologic point of view, the primary cause of death and the age of the decedent are the most pertinent. In many countries, personal identification numbers are also registered that not only provide unique identification of each person, but also the possibility to link different registers containing that number automatically. (To be discussed later in this Chapter.)

The broader the category, the better the reliability of the registered *cause of death*. The fact of death can always be accepted as a certainty. In addition, the major categories of cause of death (e.g., cancer, cardiovascular diseases, violent deaths) are usually correctly registered. The likelihood of misclassi-

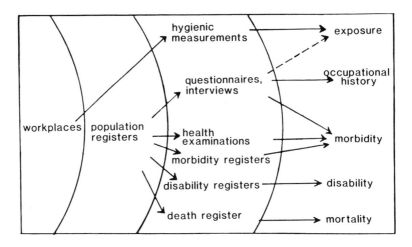

Figure 1. Flow chart showing the use of sources of information in a country with good registers.

fication increases as the diagnosis becomes more specific. For example, primary and metastatic cancers may be confused. The reliability of death registers varies from country to country. Their quality is, to some extent, related to the frequency of autopsies, but not completely, because a death certificate may be written already prior to an autopsy and not amended to include later findings. Regional variations in the frequency of autopsies within a country may also result in systematic differences in accuracy. Certain causes of death may be difficult to differentiate accurately without an autopsy, such as different causes of sudden death. Some physicians may favor coronary infarction, while others favor stroke. Locating the primary site of a cancer may also require an autopsy.

The broader the classification, the more reliable the registered cause of death.

Furthermore, different diseases are recorded in different proportions if the cause of death is due to several diseases. Cancer usually appears on a high proportion of death certificates, whereas other diseases, such as diabetes, hypertension, and pneumonia are not recorded to the same extent, even if present at the time of death. Although two or more diagnoses appear on more than half of the death certificates, only one—the primary cause of death—is usually recorded in the mortality statistics. Therefore, other diagnoses cannot be used for mortality studies.

Example 1. Suppose that mortality from prostatic cancer among workers exposed to cadmium is being investigated. Although prostatic cancer is a common secondary finding in autopsies, especially in higher age categories, only those cancers registered as the *primary cause* of death among the exposed can be used in a mortality study in order to ensure comparability with national mortality data, because secondary findings are not well recorded in national mortality statistics. However, if the data of the exposed workers are compared to an ad hoc reference group, secondary findings can also be compared (preferably as a separate category) provided the diagnostic accuracy of both groups is symmetrical.

Only the primary cause of death can be used for mortality studies if the general population is the reference.

Although the occupation is registered on the death certificate, occupational mortality cannot be studied directly from mortality registers for two main reasons. First, no satisfactory system exists for coding occupations for investigative purposes. Not even the Nordic Classification of Occupations, internationally considered to be of high quality, is ideal for this purpose. Second, the recorded occupation seldom yields complete, or even correct, information on the entire work history of the decedent. Most people have been employed in several jobs during their lifetime, and their last employment (the end occupation) often has nothing to do with possible earlier occupational risks. In addition, close relatives may report a "better" occupation than the real one. For example, the owner of a small workshop who has done all kinds of manual work himself, and who consequently may have been exposed to many chemical and physical factors, may be labeled "manager" on the death certificate. For old people the occupation is often recorded as "retired." There is usually no occupational information on those who have turned asocial at a later stage in life. Moreover, even if the occupational title would be correctly registered, occupations are such broad categories from the point of view of specific exposures that even relatively high risks would become masked if occupational titles were to be used as proxies for exposures. Therefore, mortality registers as such do not yield useful information for studying causal relations between occupational exposures and different diseases.

Death registers cannot be used as such for the study of occupational mortality.

Death registers (and also some morbidity registers) are useful in other ways, however. First, they provide data for the computation of expected numbers.

Second, they can be used to identify cases of the disease(s) under study once the study population has been defined from other sources. For example, one can define an exposed cohort from employers' records and then use the death register as a source of information on the causes of death of the deceased cohort members.

Other Morbidity Registers

National and regional morbidity registers exist in several countries. Some of these cover all causes of disease, e.g., the Finnish and Danish registers of hospital discharges, which contain, among other things, both the personal identification number and the diagnosis. In addition, many national pension institutes and sickness insurance institutions keep registers on morbidity. Such registers can be used for the study of morbidity indicators other than death, especially for diseases that are not recorded on death certificates (e.g., musculoskeletal disorders) or are incompletely recorded (e.g., diabetes). However, the quality of these registers varies. For example, the same diagnosis may have been recorded by different codes, especially if the period of interest is long. The diagnostic accuracy of morbidity registers is also far from perfect, and varies depending on the hospital, geographic region, and so forth. Confidentiality legislation prevents or at least complicates the use of register data in many countries.

Registers of specific diseases have been set up in many countries. Cancer registers, in particular, have been useful for occupational epidemiology. All of the Nordic countries have excellent national cancer registers, most of them established more than 40 years ago. There are also cancer registers in some North American states and provinces and in a number of other European countries. A short description of the Finnish Cancer Register illustrates how such a source of information can be used in the epidemiologic study of work-related cancer.

Example 2. The Finnish Cancer Register was founded in 1952. Registration is based on reports from hospitals, primary health care centers, pathological laboratories and private practitioners. On the average, five different reports are received for each patient. Together with mandatory reporting from 1961 on, this multiple reporting guarantees virtually 100% coverage, even though a tendency for more neglectful reporting has become evident recently. Quality control studies have also shown that the diagnostic accuracy is good—even better than that of the national mortality register as far as the primary site is concerned.[3,6]

Personal identification is based on the personal identification number; the register also contains data on occupation, domicile, date of death, and cause of death. Data on the tumor includes primary site, date of diagnosis, how the diagnosis was made, histology, and information on therapy. An experienced pathologist checks all diagnoses and classifies them according to primary site. More than 14,000 cases are reported each year. The Cancer Register publishes a booklet called "Cancer Incidence in Finland" annually. The Registry has had a central role in the development of both general and occupational cancer epidemiology in the whole country. It has published its own occupational cancer surveys and has, in addition, contributed to nearly all studies done in Finland on occupational cancer epidemiology.

With the help of the Cancer Register, not only can cancer mortality but also *cancer incidence* be studied. An incidence study is informative especially when the fatality of the cancer type is low. Availability of incident cases also increases the numbers of cases in cohort studies. In case-referent studies, the possibility to use incident cases means that many patients can be located while still alive. The quality of the exposure history is usually better when obtained from the patient than from a close relative. The Cancer Register can also provide comparable expected numbers for cohort studies on cancer incidence. In case-referent studies both cancer cases and cancer referents can be drawn from the Register. Especially when the type of tumor is rare, access to all cases that have occurred in the country is a great advantage. However, confidentiality legislation prohibits contacting the patients or their relatives through the use of register information; the contact must come through the hospital that has treated the patient. This regulation has caused much extra work.

In cohort studies, incident cancer cases can be identified from a cancer register. In case-referent studies both cases and cancer referents can be drawn from the register.

Some countries, among them Denmark, Finland, and Sweden, have registers on *congenital malformations*. Even though notification is mandatory, the coverage of these registers is far weaker than that of the cancer registers. The fact that minor malformations are not reported often enough is one problem. In addition, some malformations are diagnosed some months after birth. The Nordic registers have been used for many studies on work-related causes of congenital malformations.

Many countries have registers for *occupational accidents*. They vary from country to country with regard to coverage, type of information registered, and severity of accidents included (e.g., some countries record minor accidents, others only accidents resulting in sick leave). Internationally, only fatal accident rates are comparable. In some countries, for example, Denmark, Finland, and Sweden, national registers on *work-related diseases* are kept. The diagnostic accuracy varies from one disease to another, and the work-relatedness of the reported disease may often be open to dispute. Both under- and overreporting occurs. The quality of these registers is not very good, and their use in epidemiologic research is problematic.

Many countries have national or regional registers on many other diseases. Some of them are more, while others are less potentially work-related. These include registers on, for example, tuberculosis, stroke, coronary infarctions, and renal disease. Their potential use for epidemiologic research varies depending on their quality, the confidentiality legislation, and so forth.

POPULATION REGISTERS

In occupational epidemiology, population registers are mainly used for tracing persons who have dropped out of a follow-up or for locating cases and referents in population-based case-referent studies. Population registers contain personal identification numbers and can, therefore, be combined with other registers. However, their quality and accessibility vary greatly between different countries. If population registers are weak, or if their use for research purposes is restricted, surrogate methods for tracing persons must be used. These include the use of telephone directories, credit card agencies, parish registers, and even private detective agencies. Obviously, such sources are not ideal. Therefore the success of the follow-up of cohorts can be as low as 90% or even less in some countries, whereas 97 to 98% is considered to be the lowest acceptable rate in the Nordic countries.

A *census* is a periodical count of the whole population in a country. Several demographic data, including occupation and industrial branch, are usually registered. Although rather crude, census data have sometimes been linked to later morbidity data, for example, census data from 1970 with cancer data from 1980.

In several countries local population registers, for example, parish registers, are collected and kept as central population registers.

EXPOSURE REGISTERS

If exposure is broadly defined, employers' records, registers of occupational groups (e.g., physicians, dentists, bricklayers, and divers), and military records can be considered exposure registers. In some countries, sales and customs records are kept on toxic compounds, and exposed populations can be found from companies listed as users.

In some countries, among them Denmark and Finland, the national institutes of occupational health keep registers on all hygienic measurements they perform. For example, the Finnish institute visits about 4000 workplaces each year, and records of all the measurements are stored. These exposure measurements, although by no means representative, have been repeatedly used to document and quantify exposure, especially in case-referent studies on occupational cancer.

Convention 139 of the International Labour Organization (ILO), concerning the prevention and control of occupational hazards caused by carcinogens, had, by the end of 1990, been ratified by more than 20 countries, among them Denmark, the Federal Republic of Germany, Finland, Hungary, Italy,

Japan, Norway, Sweden, Switzerland, and Yugoslavia, but not Canada and the United States. The ratifying countries have committed themselves to establishing nationwide registers of *workers exposed to carcinogens*. However, thus far, only Finland has done so, (in 1979[2]).

The objective of the ILO is to promote the prevention of occupational cancer because it is assumed that an employer would prefer to exchange a carcinogenic substance for a noncarcinogenic one to avoid being listed in the register. Research was not the primary purpose. The quality of the exposure data cannot be anything but inexact and crude as the information is collected routinely from thousands of employers. Moreover, because the evidence of carcinogenicity must be strong before a chemical becomes listed, such registers have only limited use in the epidemiologic research on occupational cancer. At least it is dificult to conceive how they could aid the identification of new carcinogens. At best, they may help find exposed subjects for cohort studies, especially when the exposure is scattered, for example, occurring in many small workplaces.

REGISTER LINKAGE

Register linkage studies have become more and more common due to the increasing availability of computerized registers for which the identification of registered individuals is based on their unique personal identification number. As already mentioned, information gathered at an earlier census can be combined with information from the cancer register for the purpose of studying cancer morbidity by occupation. In a similar way, the mortality of occupational cohorts can be followed through linkage of the cohort to a national or regional register of causes of death. However, this method of studying the morbidity of large populations poses several problems.

Because registers are usually set up and maintained for administrative, not scientific, purposes, register data have limitations from the point of view of epidemiologic research. Although they are useful for computing expected numbers, for identifying "cases" in cohort studies, and for selecting cases and referents in case-referent studies and although the availability of good population registers greatly facilitates the locating of people, mechanical use of register data as such for research cannot be recommended. Most register data are crude and misclassification common. The quality control of data from large populations (say, hundreds of thousands or even millions of people) is always more difficult than that of data from smaller populations (say, cohorts comprising some thousands of subjects). No register, however computerized, can be better than the basic data input. Usually the errors weakening the quality of register data are nonsystematic, that is, random, in character. Such errors do not lead to falsely positive conclusions. In other words, they do not give the illusion of an effect when there actually is none. Instead, the effect of random errors, be it crudeness of the data or nondifferential misclassification, is negative, and therefore it *masks a true effect* (see Chapters 5 and

8). Such effect-masking hinders the effective use of register linkage in epidemiologic research.

Register linkage is too crude a method for etiologic research.

Another problem arising from the linkage of large materials is that even very small group differences give low p-values. Such differences are usually of no biological significance, and the interpretation of the statistical significance must be cautious indeed. Another problem is the so-called multisignificance phenomenon, which is described in Chapter 9. Many statistically significant differences arise by definition whenever many comparisons are made without prior hypothesis. For example, $p = 0.05$ is so defined that one out of 20 comparisons is statistically significant. The interpretation of such ''nonsense significances'' is difficult, and both the researcher and the reader of the article must exert sound judgment. The multisignificance phenomenon has received much attention; however, the masking of true effects is probably more serious in linkage studies than possible wrong judgments made from small p-values devoid of meaning. If the effect is not visible from the data, it goes totally unnoticed, while the meaning of p-values can always be disputed.

Systematic errors may also occur. Examples of such systematic errors are regional over- or underreporting and differential preferences of certain code numbers of the International Classification of Diseases. Systematic errors may also occur in the registration of occupational titles. Because even small systematic errors result in low p-values, one must indeed be cautious when interpreting statistical significances obtained from the linkage of large registers.

Because registers kept for administrative and other nonscientific purposes are less suited for epidemiologic research, it is sometimes tempting to utilize modern computer technology for establishing so-called scientific registers. However, before making such a decision, one should be aware of the costs involved, especially in the data collection and quality assurance process. One should also know exactly for what purpose the data are going to be used. (It is not enough that ''they might prove useful in the future''.) It is especially the lack of detailed data that hampers the scientific use of administrative registers. In order to be better, a ''scientific'' register should record details that are not collected by routine in administrative registers. It is the very gathering of such detailed data that is expensive and time-consuming. In addition, the quality control of many items is expensive. After the quality control, the data must be computerized, and the register must be kept up to date. All this requires much work, and these efforts may be wasted if the plans for the future use of the register are diffuse.

The storage of basic data in an uncomputerized form or, if they are stored in a computer anyway, in their original format, is sometimes a recommendable alternative. They must, however, be so recorded that possible future data processing is easy. If good research ideas are generated and the data exist, it is the researcher's task to process them in the way his or her project requires.

Sometimes it may be difficult to decide what type of data is worthwhile to store for future use. This decision must be made separately in each case. (It must also be remembered that confidentiality legislation may restrict the storage of personal data.) However, systematic collection and storage of exposure data is always recommended because the lack of such data has weakened many otherwise sound epidemiologic investigations.

Exposure data should be kept for future use, but they should not necessarily be stored in a computerized form.

In summary, the most severe weakness of mechanical register linkage studies is the tendency for true effects to become masked. The easy availability of computers and computerized registers has made both the use and misuse of linkage studies much easier than before. There is no magic trick that transforms basic data from poor to good only through the act of computerization. Therefore one must, in general, regard linkage studies with caution, although some exceptions have proved that such studies can provide useful information if refinement of the data is possible (e.g., Reference 4). Etiologic problems, in particular require well-designed and well-conducted ad hoc studies. Crude linkage studies do not solve such problems. Experienced epidemiologists know this well; uncritical advocates for linkage studies usually represent other branches of research.

Mechanical linkage of registers seldom gives useful etiologic data. Register data are crude, inexact, and usually gathered for other purposes.

CONFIDENTIALITY

Problems related to confidentiality legislation have already been mentioned many times in this chapter. It is regrettable but true that such legislation is great obstacle for epidemiologic research in many countries, among then France, Germany, and, to some extent, Italy. It restricts or at least complicate epidemiologic research to some extent in many other countries, for example, Sweden, Norway, Denmark, the United States, Great Britain, and, recently, also Finland. The legislation varies from country to country. Sometimes the delivery of identifiable personal data is completely prohibited, and sometimes there is only the demand that the identification must be removed as soon as the data have been processed. The legislation also governs the storage of register data, such as stating who can have access and who is responsible. In some countries the data obtained from a register or collected by some other method for a research project must be destroyed after a certain period of time, or as soon as they have been used for the (research) purpose for which they were obtained.

Although legislation that is too rigid is indeed an obstacle to epidemiologic research, thereby indirectly hurting those who were intended to benefit from the legislation, epidemiologists must understand the public concern for the protection of personal integrity. There are numerous examples of misuse of register data worldwide, and it must be accepted that the legislation has come to stay. Therefore, epidemiologists must learn to live with these restrictions, although they complicate the execution of epidemiologic research and create much extra bureaucratic work. Those entering an epidemiologic project must thus familiarize themselves with the legislation in their country.

The practical consequences of the legislation on the research protocol should also be considered when a project is planned. First, one should consider thoroughly what data are essential for the study so that the gathering of unnecessary data can be avoided. This point is especially important whenever so-called sensitive data are concerned. As soon as the data analysis has been completed, the material should be made anonymous by removal of the personal identification. If possible, anonymous data should be used in all data analyses. The numbers of people having access to the material should be restricted to the minimum necessary for the conduction of the study. Whenever confidential data are being collected, for example, with questionnaires, the returned forms should be addressed to one person, who is responsible for keeping them confidential, not to an institution. The storage of the data can be important in case a follow-up is planned or the data are needed later for a check of confounding, which might have been overlooked when the study was carried out or even published. In some countries, storage requires permission from the register inspection authorities. In any case, the data must be stored to ensure that access to the material is impossible for unauthorized persons.

EXPOSURE DATA

In etiologic epidemiology, the quality of the exposure information must be at least as good as the information concerning the outcome variables. Unfortunately, this self-evident fact has, until recently, been poorly appreciated by the medically trained minds of most occupational epidemiologists. Instead, they have traditionally concentrated their efforts on securing accurate data on the disease under study, which, of course, is important, but which may be wasted effort if the demand for equally good exposure data is neglected. As long as occupational epidemiology was preoccupied with identifying effects of strong hazards, even crude exposure data were sufficient. Today, when interest has switched to the unveiling of more subtle effects, such as those caused by low levels of exposure or of weak carcinogens, the demands for detailed and accurate exposure data have grown substantially. The growing importance of quantitative epidemiology, not the least for risk assessment, also stresses the need for exposure information of higher quality. Many otherwise sound epidemiologic investigations have failed to provide useful data for the very reason that poor exposure information has led to masking, or at least to an underestimate, of the effect of interest.

It must be admitted that sometimes satisfactory exposure information plainly does not exist. This problem is especially familiar to cancer epidemiologists, whose period of interest spans decades back in time. Some of the plants in which the subjects worked may have ceased to exist, and others may have kept no records at all of past exposures. In such situations there is little to do. However, in other instances, at least some kind of past exposure data can be found, or at least some proxies for exposure can be constructed. If the focus of interest does not go very far back in time, or whenever present or even future exposure is relevant, it is indeed possible to secure useful data on exposure. This process usually requires the inclusion of a skilled hygienist, or, alternatively, of some other expert if the exposure is not chemical or physical, in the research team. Fortunately such practice has recently become more common.

Measures of Chemical Exposure

Exposure data have many dimensions. They are all important to consider in epidemiologic studies. From the point of view of providing information on individual exposure, different types of exposure information can be hierarchically ranked as follows:

1. Biological measurements* (blood, urine, alveolar air, etc.)
2. Air samples collected from the breathing zone (sampled with portable samplers)
3. Area sampling by stationary samplers
4. Categorization of the subject's exposure after evaluation by a hygienist, considering work area, type of work, and occupational title
5. Dichotomization into "exposed" and "unexposed"

---

*Biological measurements are valid only if they are representative. They may also be used as proxies of other exposures, for example, if there is mixed exposure and biological monitoring tests exist for one component only (not necessarily the most toxic one).

Class 4 and especially class 5 are too crude to be used in quantitative research, although they can be used in qualitative studies. Biologic samples, when representative and correctly measured, are the best for evaluating the total (occupational plus nonoccupational) exposure of individuals or groups of people.

Collection of Exposure Data

Exposure surveys can be regular or occasional. They may cover one work site, one plant, or the industry of a whole geographic area. Usually the epidemiologist has to use existing data, that is, data already gathered for some other purpose than a certain study, but sometimes an exposure survey can be made to serve the purposes of a particular study. If this is the case, the strategy of data acquisition can be planned accordingly. Ideally the exposure information should be gathered to provide at least the following data:

- Type of exposure(s). Is there one or more exposing agents; are there relevant impurities?
- Duration of the exposure(s), preferably spanning the whole work life of each subject
- The calendar time of the exposure(s) and the relation both to the age of each subject and to the outbreak of the disease
- Intensity and type of the exposure(s)

The *quality* of the exposures should be registered in detail, because synergistic, additive, or sometimes even antagonistic effects may occur. Technical products often contain toxicologically relevant impurities. Very evidently, the *intensity* of the exposure should be known. In qualitative studies this knowledge relates to the power of the study to detect an existing effect, and in quantitative studies it is relevant for exposure-response considerations. The *duration* of the exposure is important for the same reasons. The *type* of exposure can be relevant when peaks are suspected of causing the effect, such as some neurotoxic effects of solvents. In other cases, a steady, long-standing exposure may be biologically more important, for example, certain dust exposures. Peak exposures are also important to register if the objective of the study is to provide scientific data for the setting of hygienic standards. For example, the American threshold limit values and many other national standards may have different limits for peak exposures and 8-h average exposures. Also, for the same reasons, skin exposure should be noted for agents that cross the cutaneous barrier.

The *calendar time* of the exposure(s) is relevant when diseases having a long latency period are studied. In addition, the level of occupational hygiene in general has improved in many countries and the work methods have changed substantially over the years. Recent exposure may thus be quite another matter than the same type of exposure, say, 20 years ago. Finally, the *nature* of the exposure data (i.e., on what type of information they are based) is relevant for judging their representativeness and validity.

Provided that sufficiently detailed data exist, *exposure indices* can be constructed, that are based on the duration and intensity of exposure. Even if the data are inexact, coarse *exposure categories* can be formed in the same manner. However, detailed indices derived from crude exposure data are meaningless and should not be attempted.

Accurate and detailed exposure data are important, especially in quantitative studies.

Proxies for Exposure Data

Unfortunately, retrospective exposure measurements, if they exist, are usually deficient. Missing measurements can, of course, not be compensated for. However, as a surrogate for past exposure, present levels can usually be measured, and past exposure levels can be approximated on the basis of these data, supplemented by estimates obtained from interviews of the employer, foremen, and older workers. In addition, earlier measurements made in plants of similar type can be used as proxies. An experienced hygienist can then assess past exposure by combining all these sources of information. Additional information can, perhaps, be obtained from the cumulative use of chemicals at the plant in question. Moreover, the calendar time of major changes in the process, or of major hygienic improvements such as the installation of exhaust ventilation systems, have usually been recorded. However, although this kind of information can serve qualitative studies well, it rarely gives good enough estimates for quantitative purposes. Sometimes old conditions can be simulated, for example, through the closing of the exhaust ventilation system. However, usually so many other changes have been made over the years that merely shutting off the ventilation does not give an accurate simulation of past conditions.

Job-Exposure Matrices

In the 1980s, a new approach to exposure assessment was developed. It has been named the *job-exposure matrix* (JEM). The JEM is a cross-tabulation of occupational titles and related exposures. With this approach, the occupational history can be "translated" mechanically into an exposure history, usually with the aid of a computer (see Example 11, Chapter 4). Although the method is quick, the quality of the exposure data is fairly coarse because exposures vary greatly within an occupation. The JEM classifies everyone belonging to the same occupational category as either exposed or unexposed, and this process inevitably causes misclassification with regard to the true exposure situation. The use of general (e.g., national) exposure matrices is therefore recommended only for the preliminary analysis of large materials, and even then only high risks can be revealed. In smaller studies, it is better to construct ad hoc matrices for each plant and each period of calendar time.

The occupational history can be translated into an exposure history with the aid of job-exposure matrices (JEM). This method is best suited for the preliminary analysis of large materials.

Now that the first enthusiasm has subsided, one can say that the JEM is a useful tool, although only one of several methods, for assessing exposure indirectly. Its most important use lies in the screening of large materials, mostly for qualitative purposes. For quantitative purposes more specific methods are needed. The construction of a good JEM not only requires competence in occupational hygiene but also a considerable input of manpower. If the JEM method reveals elevated risks, the finding should be scrutinized further by means of more refined exposure assessments.

Multiple Exposures

One of the most difficult problems in exposure assessment is the extremely common occurrence of multiple exposures. Most workers are simultaneously exposed to a variety of chemical agents at work; in addition, there may be exposure to noise, vibration, and other physical factors. Exposures during leisure-time activities are also complicating factors. This is not even the whole problem. During their worklives most people hold several jobs, each with its own pattern of exposure, which, in addition, changes over time as industrial processes develop. Obtaining an exposure history of such complex experience is often a formidable task. Moreover, making sense of that complex pattern is equally difficult. For example, a recent study analyzed the work patterns and exposure profiles of 774 employees in two large chemical plants. The results showed that the transfers of the employees did not follow any predictable pattern, that over 41% of the chemicals identified were found in multiple areas, and that workers exposed to one chemical were also likely to be exposed to other toxic materials.[5] This analysis concerned one employer only! The authors recommended the use of both work area and chemical-specific exposure measures or some refinement of a JEM approach, but even so etiologic studies may often fail to pinpoint the specific agent causing the disease of interest. Such problems are obstacles especially when the time relationship between exposure and effect is long, such as is the case for work-related cancer.

Nonchemical Exposures

In occupational epidemiology "exposures" are often considered to be the same as chemical exposures, but there are many other conditions in the work environment that can be of significance in the etiology of work-related diseases. Physical factors such as noise, vibration, heat, cold, or radiation form one important category of exposures with potential deleterious health effects. However, the problems related to the measurement of such factors are similar to those related to chemical factors and therefore do not warrant specific comments. Very different problems of measurement are encountered for physical and mental loads. These problems are presented in Chapter 6 and are, therefore, not introduced here.

Masking of True Effects by Crude Exposure Data

It should be stressed once more that coarseness and inaccuracy of exposure data result in *random errors*, which in a *qualitative* study, tend to mask or at least decrease true differences *between* groups (i.e., they lead to falsely negative results). In a *quantitative* study they flatten the slopes of the exposure–effect and exposure–response relationships. When differences *within* a group are being scrutinized, this flattening effect leads to overestimation of the actions of low doses and underestimation of those of high doses (Figure 2).

Figure 2, as well as the considerations presented in this context, illustrate how disastrous poor exposure data can be for the sensitivity of a study. Therefore, no efforts should be spared to provide good exposure data. Correct classification of the subjects into appropriate exposure categories is also important. If some subjects cannot be classified due to a lack of or insufficient data, it is best to leave them out, because the inclusion of such subjects would only lead to a higher than necessary proportion of wrongly classified individuals, thus weakening the study.

INDICATORS OF MORBIDITY

Measurements

There are two types of measurement scales: categorical and continuous. With a categorical variable the measured entity is placed in two or more discrete categories, such as dead/alive or high/medium/low. If there are two categories, the variable is said to be dichotomous; if there are more, it is termed polychotomous. The polychotomous scale can either be nominal or ordinal. In a nominal scale, the categories are unrelated, for example, birth district, occupation, and marital status, while the categories in an ordinal scale are related, for example, never smokers, light smokers, moderate smokers, heavy smokers, and ex-smokers.

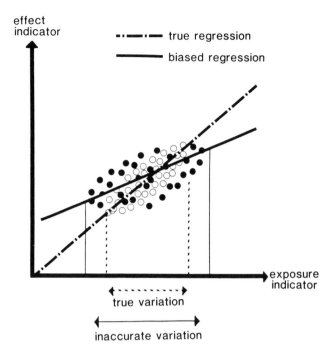

Figure 2. Inaccuracy of the exposure data increases the scatter on the horizontal axis and leads to a flattening of the slope of the exposure-effect curve, whereby effects of high doses become underestimated and those of low doses overestimated.

Continuous variables are expressed by numbers having equal successive intervals. Blood pressure, serum cholesterol level, vital capacity, and body weight are examples of continuous variables. However, a continuous variable can be categorized, for example, body weight 50 to 59, 60 to 69, and 70 to 79 kg.

Measurements can vary both because of true biological variation and because of errors in the measurement itself. Biological variation means the normally occurring variability between and within individuals. For example, even people of the same age have different blood pressures, blood counts, and serum cholesterol levels. Another type of biological variation takes place within the same individual as a function of time, for example, variations in blood pressure due to time of day, physical activity, or mental stress. Biological variation can be controlled if one ensures that the study groups are large enough and the measurements are standardized (e.g., by requiring 8 h of fasting in a supine position before the measurement, or by always doing the measurement at the same time of day, depending on the type of variation to be controlled).

Errors of measurement can be either random or systematic. They are described in Chapter 5.

"Hardness" of the Indicator

Measurements vary with regard to reliability. Certain events, such as death, are subject to no ambiguity, and also many measurements performed with modern and sophisticated equipment are highly reliable. Such measurements are usually referred to as "hard." Less reliable measurements, such as reports of subjective symptoms and other anamnestic information, are analogously called "soft." Many superficially looking hard measurements can, in fact, be rather soft. For example, causes of death may be wrongly diagnosed, and X-ray films may be misread. Likewise, anamnestic data need not be unreliable. Several types can be valid, for example, the number of one's own children or reports of long periods of employment.

One could be misled to think that hard parameters should always be preferred because of their better reliability. This is not true. The optimum hardness of a parameter depends on the nature of the problem. Death is such a crude measure that a mortality study can reveal only the most severe health hazards. Many diseases, such as musculoskeletal disorders, mental diseases, and eczemas, are not registered on the death certificates. Even ultimately fatal diseases, such as coronary heart disease, have earlier and/or milder stages, whose study may deepen the understanding of the relation between a certain exposure and the disease. One can say that while hard indicators of morbidity are, in general, more reliable, soft indicators are more sensitive. Sensitivity can be more desirable than reliability in many instances, if the price of the latter property is loss of power to detect deleterious properties of the exposure in question.

Hard indicators are usually more reliable, soft indicators more sensitive. The nature of the problem determines the optimum hardness.

Example 3. The Finnish carbon disulfide study[1,7] which is presented in several examples in this book, used a wide range of morbidity indicators, namely, coronary death, nonfatal infarctions, symptoms of angina, "coronary" electrocardiographic changes at rest and after exercise, blood pressure, and serum lipids. The most prominent effect was that coronary mortality was increased by 4.7-fold. (See Example 6, Chapter 4.) Several other indicators also showed an effect of carbon disulfide exposure, such as symptoms of angina ($\widehat{RR}$ = 2.2) and "coronary" electrocardiographic changes ($\widehat{RR}$ = 1.4). However, hindsight has shown that the softer indicators did not add much to the information given by the hardest [death from coronary heart disease (CHD)]. The preventive program that was initiated was certainly influenced more by the mortality data than by the milder manifestations of morbidity. The costs of registering mortality were only a minor part of the total costs of the project. After the results of the first 5 years of follow-up had been analyzed, only mortality was followed for the next 10 years.

Questionnaires and Interviews

Many milder health effects or symptoms, such as fatigue, dizziness, nausea, pain, mucosal irritation, and paresthesias, can only be studied through the use of self-administered questionnaires or structured interviews. These methods are also frequently used for gathering data on past exposures and lifestyle variables. These are soft methods, and their use poses problems typical of soft measurements.

Self-administered questionnaires are usually highly structured and specifically designed for a certain study. The quality of the information obtained depends strongly on how well the questions have been formulated. It is recommended to test all questionnaires on a sample of respondents before their use on a larger scale so that their functions can be determined and poor questions improved. It is also advisable to make provision for later contact by telephone or mail so that unclear or deficiently reported issues can be resolved. In questionnaire studies, nonresponse is always a problem. One should therefore repeat the mailing at least twice; even so, the response rate may be as low as 70 to 75%. (Repeated mailing is not possible if the replies are returned unidentified, a matter to ponder thoroughly during the planning of the survey.) Nonresponse is a problem because those who do not return the questionnaire may differ systematically in relevant aspects from those who return it. If possible, at least the most relevant differences between respondents and nonrespondents (e.g., social structure, smoking status) should be checked by some other method, for example, a telephone interview to a sample of the nonrespondents. However, nonresponse is not necessarily systematic, at least not in all respects, and therefore does not inevitably cause bias. For example, in case-referent studies inquiring into exposure history, there is rarely reason to assume that cases and referents respond in a systematically different manner, but the problem remains that one can never be sure of the reasons for nonresponse.

Interviews overcome some of the mentioned problems, but they are more time-consuming and therefore more expensive. They can be carried out either in hospitals, in personal visits, or by telephone. Usually the nonresponse rate is lower in interview studies than in studies using self-administered questionnaires, but the interviewer, if not properly trained and careful, may introduce another type of problem, so-called observer bias, which is described in Chapter 5.

Sensitivity and Specificity

Every population is composed of individuals who either have a certain disease or are free of it. By measuring certain indicators of this disease, one tries to classify the individuals correctly, that is, diseased persons as sick and healthy persons as healthy (with regard to the specific disease). This is an important issue in scientific epidemiologic studies, and also in health care practice, in which screening programs are run to detect various work-related and other diseases.

If the disease indicator is good at identifying sick persons, it is said to be *sensitive*. Sensitivity is the property of giving a positive result when the disease is present (i.e., the probability of detecting that disease). Hence,

$$\text{Sensitivity} = \frac{\text{diseased persons classified as sick}}{\text{truly diseased persons}}$$

If, on the other hand, the disease indicator is good at identifying healthy persons, it is said to be *specific*. Specificity is the property of giving a negative result when the disease is absent, that is, the probability of the test correctly classifying people as healthy (with regard to that specific disease). Hence,

$$\text{Specificity} = \frac{\text{healthy persons classified as healthy}}{\text{truly healthy persons}}$$

However, no test is perfect, and therefore some healthy people may be classified as sick. Such errors of classification are called *false positives*. Likewise, some sick persons may be classified as being free from the disease. Such errors of classification are called *false negatives*. A sensitive indicator easily identifies true positives (i.e., sick persons), but it also tends to give falsely positive results. Correspondingly, a specific test identifies correctly those without the disease, but it also tends to give falsely negative results.

A sensitive indicator may give falsely positive results, and a specific indicator falsely negative ones.

Sensitivity and specificity are usually interrelated,(i.e., the higher the sensitivity, the lower the specificity, and vice versa). Depending on the nature of the problem, either high sensitivity or high specificity should be chosen; both properties can usually not be achieved.

Screening programs are usually based on the use of relatively simple tests, whose sensitivity and specificity should be known. If the disease that is being screened for is severe (e.g., cancer), sensitive tests are preferred. This choice, unfortunately, also tends to result in a high proportion of false positives, which can lead to expensive and cumbersome further diagnostic procedures. In addition, those falsely classified as positive may experience anxiety. However, underdiagnosing severe diseases would probably be an even greater disadvantage, and, for this reason, sensitivity is usually preferred over specificity if the disease is potentially serious. The situation is different when screening for milder diseases, such as early diabetes. In such instances, the border for "positivity" is usually placed rather high on the continuous scale of blood glucose values, so that not too many false positives appear. Many falsely positive results would easily overload the diagnostic capacity of the health center or hospital. The price for high specificity is that some incipient case of diabetes may wrongly be classified as healthy and thereby escape early detection. However, a diagnostic delay of 1 or 2 years probably does not affect the course of adult diabetes.

The higher the sensitivity, the lower the specificity; the higher the specificity, the lower the sensitivity.

In screening programs, the sensitivity and specificity of a test also depend on the prevalence of the disease (P). The positive predictivity (Pred) of a test can be expressed in the following way:

$$\text{Pred} = \frac{P \times \text{sensitivity}}{P \times \text{sensitivity} + (1 - P) \times (1 - \text{specificity})}$$

Example 4. Suppose that P = 20% and that both the sensitivity and the specificity are 99% (which is unusual). Then,

$$\text{Pred} = \frac{0.2 \times 0.99}{0.2 \times 0.99 + (1 - 0.2) \times (1 - 0.99)} = 96.1$$

However, if P = 1%, the predictivity drops to 50%. If the sensitivity and the specificity are 80% (which still is far from poor) and if P = 20%, the predictivity is again 50%, but if P = 1%, it is only 3%.

Example 4 illustrates that screening for rare diseases is inefficient and that tests having low sensitivity and specificity are of little value in screening programs. This reasoning also applies to epidemiologic research in the sense that the empirical parameters used as indicators of morbidity should be selected with both specificity and sensitivity in mind. If both properties cannot be combined, the nature of the problem must decide whether sensitivity or specificity is to be preferred.

Specificity has another dimension, however. A test can be specific either to a certain *exposure* or to a certain *organ system*. For example, lead exposure causes (apart from elevated blood lead values) certain well-defined disturbances in heme synthesis, for example, increased excretion of δ-aminolevulinic acid in the urine. On the other hand, *exposure-nonspecific* effects belong to the character of many work-related diseases. One example is coronary infarction and exposure to carbon disulfide. Another example is chronic bronchitis and exposure to dust, while a third is polyneuropathy and exposure to certain solvents. Although exposure-nonspecific, all of these manifestations are *organ-specific*, coronary infarction to the heart, bronchitis to the airways, and polyneuropathy to the peripheral nervous system. There are also *organ-nonspecific* symptoms such as fatigue, low-back pain (muscles, intravertebral discs, ligaments, bony structures, visceral organs), and breathlessness (heart, lungs, anemia). Both specific and nonspecific effects can be used in epidemiologic research, but the more nonspecific the manifestation, the greater the need for a valid reference group.

REFERENCES

1. Hernberg, S., T. Partanen, C. H. Nordman, and P. Sumari. "Coronary heart disease among workers exposed to carbon disulphide," *Br. J. Ind. Med.* 27:313 (1970).
2. Herva, A. "The Finnish register of employees occupationally exposed to carcinogens, *Proceedings of the International Symposium on Prevention of Occupational Cancer, Helsinki*, 1981 Geneva: International Labour Office, 1982. (Occupational Safety and Health Series, No. 46), 569.
3. Lehtonen, M. and E. Saxen. "Syöpäkuolintodistusten luotettavuus Suomessa (Reliability of cancer death certificates in Finland)," *Duodecim* 88:1100 (1972).
4. Malker, H. S. R., J. K. McLaughlin, B. K. Malker, B. J. Stone, J. A. Weiner, J. L. E. Erickson, and W. J. Blot. "Occupational risk for pleural mesothelioma in Sweden, 1961-79," *J. Natl. Cancer Inst.* 74:61 (1985).
5. Ott, M.G., M. J. Teta, and H. L. Greenberg. "Assessment of exposure to chemicals in a complex work environment," *Am. J. Ind. Med.* 16:617 (1989).
6. Teppo, L. "Suomen syöpärekisteri (The Finnish Cancer Registry), *Sosiaalivakuutus* 7-8:218 (1980).
7. Tolonen, M., S. Hernberg, M. Nurminen, and K. Tiitola. "A follow-up study of coronary heart disease in viscose rayon workers exposed to carbon disulphide, *Br. J. Ind. Med.* 32:1 (1975).

CHAPTER 4

Epidemiologic Study Designs and Their Applications in Occupational Medicine

INTRODUCTION

The first step in the planning of an epidemiologic study is the definition of the problem. Before doing anything else, researchers must ensure that they have a clear view of the problem at the abstract-general level: they must conceptualize it. At the conceptual level a qualitative problem takes the form of "does X cause Y?," and it is further refined by the specification of the circumstances under which this process may or may not happen. A quantitative problem deals with "how much will a certain amount of exposure to X affect the risk of Y?" As soon as, but not before, the researchers know exactly what scientific problem the study should address, they can define the empirical occurrence variables of the exposure and the effect that will be measured. For example, at the conceptual level the problem could take the form "does carbon disulfide cause coronary heart disease?" This question implies that carbon disulfide is a causal risk factor of coronary heart disease, one of its many causes, and, if it really is, that the cardiotoxic effect of carbon disulfide is "general." Therefore, the effect found in a particular study would not be confined to that study population, but would apply to other similarly exposed populations as well. However, the scientific generalization cannot be made until a particular setting has been studied empirically, that is, a certain population, certain exposure conditions, and certain indicators of the disease. One could, for example, measure the air concentrations of carbon disulfide in a particular plant during A years and select one or more indicators of the disease, such as clinical coronary infarction, to be measured in an exposed and reference population over a period of B years. Not only the occurrence relation itself, meaning the parameters of exposure and outcome, but also potential confounders and effect modifiers (see Chapter 5) must be defined and plans made for their measurement.

Considerations regarding the population whose morbidity experience makes up the study base should involve its eligibility criteria, its aimed size, and how the exposure, potential confounders, and effect-modifying factors are distributed. The timing of the study should define both the time period during which information on morbidity has accrued, say, the past 30 years, and the calendar time during which that information will be collected, say, the next year. Plans should also be made for securing valid observations. Finally, one should decide whether the information will be gathered from the whole study population (census design), or from a sample of it (case-referent design), and how large a population will be needed to provide enough information for correct conclusions regarding the compared disease incidences. It should be stressed that researchers are interested in the scientific facts, not the particular morbidity experience of the study population, which only serves as an empirical instrument for the study of the scientific "truth."

As already stressed, it is important that the researchers themselves understand the objectives of the study clearly before starting the project. The objectives should also be stated explicitly in the study protocol, not to mention the final manuscript. If the objectives are poorly defined in the mind of the researcher and on paper, the study is not likely to be good.

The objectives of a study must be stated clearly. The researcher must be able to distinguish between the conceptual and the empirical level of the problem. If the objectives are poorly conceptualized, the study has a poor prospect.

The actual setting in which the scientific problem is studied is called the *study base*,[12] which can be thought of as the morbidity experience (in relation to some exposure) of a population while it is followed in time. Thus the study base is not only a population, a number of people, but the morbidity experience of this population during a certain period of time.

The study base is the morbidity experience of a population over time.

The incidence of the disease can, depending on a number of factors discussed later in this chapter and in Chapter 5, be acquired either by examining *all* the individuals belonging to the study base population (a census = 100% sample), or the incidence can be studied by comparing, with regard to the relevant exposure, the *cases* of the disease of interest to a *sample*, either of the whole study base or of individuals free from the disease. The first approach corresponds to what has traditionally been called a *cohort design*, the second to what has been called a *case-referent* or case-control design. The sampling of the study base (the case-referent approach) can be made from either dynamic or closed populations. It is important to realize that a census and a sampling approach, for example, a census design and a case-referent study within the cohort base, are two alternative approaches to extracting scientific matter from the same study base, not completely contrasting study designs, as has been believed earlier. Matters related to feasibility, efficiency, and validity usually determine which approach is the best in each particular situation.

If the morbidity of the study population is followed over some period of time, the study is said to be *longitudinal*. However, a study can also be designed as a cross-section of the study base at a certain point in time, in which case the study has no time span. In such a *cross-sectional* design the prevalence of a disease is measured in relation to its determinants. The prevalence is a composite parameter; it depends on the incidence rate, the rate of cure, the fatality rate, and the duration of the disease. (Those not yet diseased, those cured, and those who have died are excluded from the base population.) In addition, health-selective turnover may have distorted the information contained in the prevalence rate. Prevalence studies are best suited for the study of stable diseases of long duration. They are usually descriptive and aimed at solving particularistic (time- and space-specific) problems. They often have an administrative rather than a scientific purpose (e.g., studying the prevalence of diabetics in a population with the aim of planning for resources for regular controls or surveying the prevalence of occupational lead exposure in a geographic area for the purpose of locating dangerous work conditions). While helpful in public or occupational health practice, their use is rather limited for etiologic research because of the circumstances discussed later in this chapter and in Chapter 5.

A cross-sectional study is a cross section of the study base; a longitudinal study has a time dimension.

For solving etiologic problems, a follow-up of the study base—an incidence study—is better suited than a cross section of it. The incidence of a disease is usually more informative than its prevalence, and incidence studies must be longitudinal. Many diseases, both work-related and others, do not occur suddenly, but develop during a period of time. Hence, the onset of exposure and the manifestation of the disease are separated by a time period, which may sometimes be long. Therefore, the etiologic study of such diseases requires a design in which the exposure and the outcome are measured at different points in time.

Although cross sections of the study base are usually descriptive prevalence studies, they can sometimes provide etiologic information. One example is the study of diseases with short or no latency, for example, respiratory symptoms caused by irritant gases. A cross-sectional design can also provide information on the etiology of chronic diseases, provided the exposure has been stable over time. For example, the effects of stable lead exposure on the peripheral nervous system can be studied with the current blood lead concentration as a proxy for past exposure if it is known that conditions have not changed much during the past 5 years or so. A cross-sectional morbidity study can, however, be valid only if the disease in question does not cause health-based selection out of the exposed job. For example, noise-induced hearing impairment would probably not cause much selective turnover, at least not in its milder stages, while back pain would certainly have great effects. However, in general, a longitudinal design is to be preferred for the study of etiologic problems.

Cross-sectional designs are usually descriptive prevalence studies; etiologic problems require a longitudinal design.

DESCRIPTIVE SURVEYS

Survey of the General Health of Employees

A workplace can be considered a miniature community, the health problems of which can be surveyed with epidemiologic methods. Some health problems of the employees may be work-related, but most of them are usually composed of diseases and disorders that can be present in any population. However, because interactions between work and health always occur, even diseases without any work-related etiology often affect work capacity. Hence, all diseases of employees are a concern of a comprehensive occupational health care system. Such a health care system—at least in countries where legislation does not restrict the contents of occupational health care—should provide for regular health surveillance of the personnel. An epidemiologic approach can help systematize routine occupational health care programs. Systematic surveillance programs are usually focused on specific categories of employees, chosen because of some common risk factor. The surveillance programs can, for example, be designed to:

1. Survey regularly workers exposed to known occupational health hazards
2. Examine workers coming into contact with new health hazards
3. Keep close surveillance of workers with an increased sensitivity to incur work-related diseases (e.g., elderly workers, atopics, pregnant women)
4. Identify, with the help of screening programs, those workers with exceptional risk to incur certain other diseases (e.g., coronary heart disease), in order to take preventive action
5. Diagnose employees with mild curable disorders (e.g., iron deficiency, refraction anomalies)
6. Diagnose chronic diseases which require regular control (e.g., diabetes, hypertension)

7. Identify those workers who are not suitable for certain jobs (e.g., those having allergies, chronic bronchitis, back disorders)
8. Keep those with an unhealthy life-style under closer scrutiny (e.g., heavy smokers, alcohol abusers, obese persons) in order to help them cope with their problem

Usually the resources of the occupational health care services are restricted. Therefore, the objectives of the surveillance program should be well defined in advance to ensure optimal allocation of manpower and funds. Is the aim to initiate a regular surveillance program, is it to identify high-risk individuals for control programs, is it to improve the efficiency of routine check-up programs, or is it something else?

Health surveillance programs should be focused on specific risk groups, and their objectives should be clearly defined in advance.

Equally important is the selection of sufficiently sensitive and specific tests for the screening programs (see Chapter 3). The use of "comprehensive" biochemical and other test batteries is no longer recommended, partly because of the high costs involved, partly because of the long, resource-demanding and often completely unnecessary further examinations they incur, but mostly because of their low yield in terms of disease prevention. Therefore, one should be selective, both with regard to what condition will be screened for and what tests will be used.

Example 1. Suppose storage battery workers exposed to lead are being surveyed with the aim of preventing toxic lead effects. The dose–effect relationship for various toxic effects such as hematologic changes and disturbances of nervous function are fairly well known by now. Accepting these data as reliable, it would suffice to measure regularly the concentration of lead in the blood (B–Pb), because if B–Pb remains low, say, below 40 μg/100 mL (about 2 μmol/L), it is known that no major toxic manifestations should occur. Measuring, in addition, the concentration of δ-aminolevulinic acid in the urine, would identify the most sensitive individuals. Both these tests are specific. Some physicians would consider measuring the conduction velocity in peripheral nerves, for example, once every second year. However, this test is not specific to lead, and requires special, rather sophisticated equipment (at least from the point of view of an occupational health service unit). Therefore, it is not suited for the routine surveillance of workers. If one relies on the known dose–response relationship between lead exposure, on the one hand, and peripheral nervous function impairment on the other (see Table 4, Chapter 2), no harmful effects are expected as long as the B–Pb remains below μg/100 mL. The fairly common practice of periodically examining the blood count is not worthwhile from the point of view of preventing lead poisoning because anemia is a late manifestation of lead toxicity. Furthermore, the white blood cell count is not at all affected by lead. As long as one can be sure that the B–Pb stays below the threshold level for a given toxic effect, it is irrelevant to look for that effect. However, it must be stressed that these considerations concern routine health surveillance programs, not diagnostic examinations of patients suspected of having lead poisoning.

Insensitive methods do not detect those having the disease in question, whereas nonspecific methods give too many false positive findings (see Chapter 3). A screening program is successful only if the occupational health service or, alternatively, some other health care system can handle the necessary further examinations and corrective measures (treatment, etc.) that a screening activity always results in. Likewise, if the possibilities to transfer the workers to less demanding jobs are limited or nonexistent, it is not rational to initiate activities to "identify" handicapped workers who themselves are usually perfectly well aware of their reduced work capacity. If the aim of the surveillance program is early diagnosis and prevention, the disease must indeed be preventable. At least it must be possible to improve its course. If these requirements are not met, the surveillance program may cause more harm in the form of unnecessary worry than benefit in terms of successful prevention.

Finally, all working populations have a turnover and their disease patterns change over time. Therefore surveillance programs must be planned with continuity in mind, and the health examinations should be repeated periodically. The costs can be reduced if the examinations focus on those categories of employees who are likely to be at high risk, such as those exposed to chemicals, those over 40 years of age, heavy smokers, and the like.

Observation of Morbidity in Relation to Occupation, Work Area, or Certain Exposures

Systematic health surveys of workers who are exposed to a "cocktail" of chemical agents, to strenuous work, or to some other ill-defined condition may provide the first clue that something is wrong in the workplace. Although primary prevention should be based on direct observations of the work environment, data gathered from health surveillance programs can also be used for initiating improvements in work conditions. Such a surveillance activity can rarely use hard indicators of disease. Soft parameters indicating slighter effects are better suited for this purpose. Suitable methods for occupational health care services are, for example, structured questionnaires, interviews, information from routine records, data on absenteeism, and various clinical, biochemical, and functional examinations. Because the rationale of such a medical surveillance program is to relate the findings to some factor(s) at work, the exposure (in a broad sense) must also be defined. Much consideration must be given to the choice of effect indicators. If the exposure is ill defined, there are no specific (to what?) tests. Sensitivity is, therefore, more important. If some test shows evidence of abnormality, the cause of the abnormality must next be elucidated, which means that the exposure itself should be studied. If, on the other hand, one already suspects that a certain exposure may be harmful, specificity of the effect indicator becomes important. Unfortunately, there are very few exposure-specific indicators (e.g., disturbances of the heme synthesis for lead), but the number of organ-specific indicators is greater (e.g., nerve conduction velocities for neurotoxicity, decreased forced expiratory volume for bronchial constriction, elevated serum creatinine level for renal dysfunction). In addition, less specific tests can be used at the group level (e.g., symptoms indicative of psychasthenia for solvent-exposed workers, symptoms of chronic bronchitis for workers exposed to dust). In all cross-sectional surveys one must, however, remember that health-based selection out of the exposed job leads to underestimation of the true risk.

This type of survey should not be confused with scientific research. It is rather a systematic approach to occupational health care. As stated many times before, a true scientific study usually requires a longitudinal design. Likewise, medical surveys are not the same as primary prevention, and, therefore, they are no substitute for preventive measures aimed at direct improvements in work conditions. If the level of occupational hygiene is high, medical surveillance programs aiming at the detection of work-related disorders would not be needed at all. Unfortunately, this ideal situation is rare.

Identification of Risks — Alarms

Sometimes descriptive epidemiologic observations may give the first warning of hitherto unknown occupational risks. For example, an unexpected increase in the occurrence of eczema may be the first indication of that a new, allergenic chemical has been introduced in the workplace without the plant physician having been notified. An alert plant physician can sometimes even be the first to note a completely new hazard. This actually happened in the early 1970s when two cases of an extremely rare tumor, angiosarcoma of the liver, were observed in the same chemical company among workers exposed to vinyl chloride. The clinical observation was soon corroborated by many similar case reports and also by several epidemiologic studies. Such clinical observations are easier to relate to a specific exposure if the disease is rare. However, sometimes the work-relatedness of more common manifestations of diseases can also be detected in this way. For example, epidemics of inflammatorylike respiratory disease have repeatedly alerted occupational health personnel to the occurrence of microorganisms in the ventilation air.

Nationwide Occupational Morbidity and Mortality Statistics

National statistics may sometimes give indications of occupational health risks. These indications are however suggestive only, because register data are usually too general to allow etiologic conclusions (see Chapter 3). The Registrar General in Great Britain has been comparing the mortality within occupational categories, on the basis of census data on the occupation 10 years previously, for the past two centuries.[5] Several occupational groups have shown increased mortality, for example, miners, ceramic workers, foundry workers, and cotton workers, who have had higher than expected mortality from dust-related diseases. The effect of occupation itself on several other elevated causes of death has been less clear because the effects of interrelated social and life-style factors cannot be separated. All in all, national registers are best suited as starting points for specific epidemiologic studies, not as providers of hard evidence of occupational health hazards. Etiologic studies require more detailed and accurate data than can be obtained directly from such registers.

CROSS SECTIONS OF THE STUDY BASE

In a scientific sense a cross-sectional design is a cross section of the study base, without any time dimension. Both exposure and morbidity (prevalence) are measured at the same point in time. The cross section is etiologically meaningful only if a true time relation exists between the exposure and the outcome. For example, a survey of the prevalence of silicosis among active foundry workers cannot give any information on the hazards posed by current silica dust levels, only on exposure conditions that prevailed decades ago. By contrast, the current concentration of B–Pb does explain the current level of the activity of the erythrocyte enzyme δ-aminolevulinic dehydratase. These parameters have repeatedly been shown to have a close temporal relation. Likewise, provided the exposure to lead has been constant over time, the current B–Pb can also explain cross-sectional results of nerve conduction velocity measurements. However, if there have been fluctuations, the time-weighted average B–Pb is a better exposure parameter. The study then is rather a hybrid than a pure cross section of the study base in the sense that the exposure is measured longitudinally while the outcome is measured cross-sectionally.

An etiologic cross-sectional study is meaningful only if a close time-relation exists between exposure and morbidity.

Example 2. Suppose that the issue is whether a certain exposure intensity of chlorine gas in pulp bleaching, say, the levels around the current hygienic standard, causes respiratory symptoms among the workers. For such a quantitative problem accurate exposure data are important. (It has been well known for over a century that chlorine is a potent respiratory toxin, and its potency was later well proved in World War I. From a qualitative point of view, then, such a study would be meaningless.)

Therefore, much effort must be devoted to gathering accurate and detailed exposure data from a period of, say, 1 or 2 months. A monthly average should be estimated for each worker, but also peak concentrations should be registered and used in the exposure classification. The workers could then be grouped into, say, three exposure categories, the most relevant being the one closest to the hygienic standard. Some criterion for minimum duration of exposure should also be set, for example, 1 month. An unexposed group of, say, paper machine workers, could be used as the reference group.

All the groups should then be given the same examination, for example, a standardized questionnaire on respiratory symptoms and simple lung function tests. Inquiry into smoking habits and possible exposures to other irritants should also be made. With control for such potential confounders, the respiratory symptoms and lung function tests of the different groups would then be compared. Suppose that the group exposed to the levels around the hygienic standard showed more symptoms than the reference group, and suppose that a more heavily exposed group had even more positive findings. The results would suggest that chlorine exposure was responsible for the findings (suggestion of a causal relationship) and would indicate that the current hygienic standard is too high. Such a study should preferably be repeated in another paper and pulp mill, and if the results were similar, administrative action should then be taken to lower the standard.

Although cross-sectional designs can sometimes convey etiologic information, the prevalence rate is not ideal as a measure of morbidity because of the composite nature of the prevalence. Meaningful interpretation of prevalence data presupposes knowledge of all the different components.

LONGITUDINAL DESIGNS — INTRODUCTORY REMARKS

Longitudinal studies have a time dimension. They measure the morbidity experience (incidence) of the study population during a certain period of time. The study population can either be dynamic or fixed. In both cases, the measurement can be done in different ways. If all the members of the base population are studied, one speaks of a census approach (census = 100% sample). Alternatively, the study can be designed to investigate all the cases of the disease of interest, but only a sample of the noncases. This approach is usually called a case-referent (case-control) design. The case-referent design can be applied to both dynamic population and cohort bases. Contrary to what has been conventionally believed, a census approach and a case-referent approach do not represent fundamentally different principles, only two different methods of gathering the same information from the study base.[12]

Example 3. Suppose again that the hypothesis is that exposure to carbon disulfide causes coronary infarction. The study base is defined as the follow-up until 1982 of a cohort of men exposed to carbon disulfide for at least 5 years in the period 1942 to 1967, as well as of a similarly large cohort of unexposed men, enrolled during the same time period.[8] Such a study base can be investigated in two ways. One way would be to elucidate the exposure history of all workers and to register the incidence of coronary infarction (fatal infarctions, hospitalized nonfatal infarctions) in the whole study base, whereafter the incidences in the exposed and unexposed groups would be compared.

Another approach would be to pool both groups, register all cases of coronary infarction, gather exposure data on the cases, and a sample of noncases (say, three or four per case), then compare the exposure frequencies among the cases and the referents, and finally compute an indirect risk estimate from the OR (see Chapter 2). The former approach corresponds to a census study of a cohort base, the latter to a so-called nested case-referent study (see later in this chapter). Both approaches use the same cohort base and yield, in principle, the same information.

Example 4. The same phenomenon could also be studied from a dynamic population base, namely, that of the small city of Valkeakoski, where both the plants are situated. That population could be followed for a certain time, say 10 years. One approach (a laborious one) would be to register the exposure history (especially with regard to work in the viscose rayon plant) of all Valkeakoski men of a certain age range (say, 40 to 64 years for the sake of study efficiency). Then the incidence of coronary infarction, obtained from the National Register of Deaths and the patient register of the Valkeakoski city hospital, could be calculated and the rates among the exposed (to carbon disulfide) and unexposed would be compared to yield an estimate of the RR.

Alternatively, cases of coronary infarction could be gathered from the same sources, a sample of noncases drawn from the population register of Valkeakoski, and the exposure histories of these individuals could then be compared to yield the $\widehat{OR}$. Again, the same information would be gained with the use of either approach.

One important difference between a cohort base and a dynamic population base is that cohort members who leave their employment or move must be included in the follow-up, whereas this procedure is not necessary for a dynamic population. Likewise, a cohort does not accrue new members after having been defined, whereas people continually join and leave a dynamic population. In particular, the turnover of a dynamic population may be due to the disease under study, and, if so, it causes selection bias if not accounted for. If the dynamic population is large enough, this source of bias is not so serious because much of the migration takes place within the population. However, it is not feasible to obtain a census of very large populations, and therefore one usually studies such populations by sampling, which calls for the case-referent approach. If the dynamic population is smaller (say, a small municipality or a part of a city), it is easier to study it with the census approach.

A smaller dynamic population base does not necessarily introduce selection bias in the study of general diseases but, as already pointed out, this approach is questionable whenever the population is defined on the basis of employment and work-related disorders are studied.

It is true that health-based migration may occur between municipalities (e.g., healthy people may migrate from rural to urban municipalities or move abroad), but this migration does not necessarily distort the study of general diseases. For example, the predictive value of the low-density lipoprotein level in serum on the development of coronary heart disease does not depend on whether people live in Cincinnati, Louisville or Miami, or whether they migrate between these cities.

Because of health-selective turnover, cohort bases have usually been preferred over dynamic population bases in the occupational health setting, although many case-referent studies on, for example, work-related cancer, have been based on dynamic populations. Although there are theoretically several different options for study design, validity and feasibility considerations often reduce the number of alternatives to one. In fact, when the alternatives presented in Examples 3 and 4 are compared, it is evident that the dynamic population base would have been far less efficient than the cohort base.

COHORT-BASED STUDIES

Census Studies

A cohort is designed to encompass subjects sharing a common event. That event could be the same year of birth, employment in the same company, exposure to a common agent, and so forth. In occupational medicine, the event of interest is usually a common occupational exposure. "Exposure" is to be viewed broadly. It may be a chemical or physical exposure, a physically strenuous job, shift work, or whatever condition is suspected of having effects on the morbidity of the exposed population. Occupation itself is also often viewed as the event—a proxy for exposure—for which cohorts are formed. However, occupation is a poor proxy for specific exposures. It is, therefore, not a good criterion for cohort formation unless the object of the study is to investigate the effects of the rather ill-defined joint exposures that occur in some occupations. A classic cohort study is a true census of the exposed population because everyone is followed-up and examined. However, as discussed later in this chapter, a study can also be designed as a sampling of the cohort base, and, in this instance, the cohort base is more informative if designed to comprise individuals with different exposure status, in order to provide contrasts. Such inclusion criteria differ from the classic cohort criteria according to which one focuses on individuals with greater exposure.

Apart from a qualitatively shared exposure, the eligibility for admission to a cohort of exposed subjects usually also requires fulfillment of other criteria.

COHORT STUDY

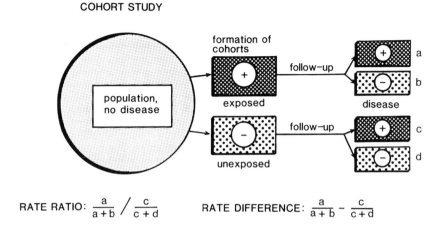

RATE RATIO: $\dfrac{a}{a+b} \Big/ \dfrac{c}{c+d}$ RATE DIFFERENCE: $\dfrac{a}{a+b} - \dfrac{c}{c+d}$

Figure 1. Design of a census study from a cohort base.

These criteria may be age, gender, minimum duration and intensity of exposure (quantitative exposure criteria), freedom from other exposures, and the like. At entrance, all cohort members should be free of the disease under study, according to the empirical set of criteria used to measure the disease.

> *Example 5.* Suppose, again, that the issue is coronary infarctions caused by carbon disulfide. Let the empirical outcome criteria be coronary deaths and hospitalized attacks of coronary infarction. Those who have had infarctions before the formation of the cohort must be excluded. However, those who may have notes of electrocardiographic changes, angina, or such in their records are not excluded, because in this example the empirical outcome parameter is clinical fatal or nonfatal infarction, not Q waves in the electrocardiogram, or a history of angina. If, on the other hand, the empirical outcome parameter would be Q waves and/or angina, then those already having these manifestations could not be accepted into the cohort. Because the occurrence of new symptoms of angina and electrocardiographic changes would be the very objective of a study designed in this way, people already having these manifestations would not be eligible.

The morbidity of an exposed cohort should preferably be compared to an ad hoc reference cohort to yield an estimate of the RR (crude or standardized). The mortality (rarely other forms of morbidity) can also be compared to age-, gender-, and time-standardized national mortality figures to yield the SMR, which indicates whether the mortality is higher or lower than "expected" (Chapter 2). If an ad hoc reference cohort is used, it should be similar to the exposed cohort in all relevant aspects, save the exposure (Figure 1). Provided it indeed is comparable, an ad hoc reference cohort gives a more valid comparison than the general population, but because it is smaller, the result of the comparison is more affected by random variation. Such variation results in a wider confidence interval for the estimate of the RR.

For reasons of efficiency, one should design the "exposed" cohort so that the members' distribution of exposure does not reflect the normally occurring near-Gaussian distribution with emphasis on the average exposure.[12] If the problem is qualitative, the issue is to determine whether a particular exposure really causes the disease of interest, in which case the estimate of the RR is over 1 in the study in question. For this purpose, one should focus on those having received the heaviest exposure instead of indiscriminantly including all the "exposed" in the cohort. However, when the qualitative aspects are known, and the interest turns to the quantitative aspects of the occurrence relation, lower exposure categories must also be included. However, again it is inefficient to design the study base indiscriminately so that it has the "right" proportions of all the exposed people (contrary to what many researchers think). Instead, one should take advice from experimental scientists and focus on the extremes, in this instance, heavily and slightly exposed individuals. This so-called two-point design is common in experimental work because of its efficiency. Unfortunately, few epidemiologists have taken advantage of its cost-saving effects. If more detailed knowledge of the occurrence relation is desirable, one can modify the two-point design into a three-point design by including a third, intermediate category. It must be admitted that the degree of exposure of each individual often becomes evident during the course of the study, lack of knowledge making exact allocations impossible at the planning stage. Even so, some crude exposure classifications are usually possible early in the course of the study. In any case, one should avoid the indiscriminate use of the entire "exposed" population (e.g., all workers in the foundry industry, all workers in a chemical company) when designing a census-type study. The exposure distribution of the study group selected by the researcher should rather approach a U-shape than the usual bell-formed Gaussian shape.[12]

It is also cost-saving to restrict the study base with regard to some other properties of the subjects. For example, if the number of subjects in one category (females, nonwhites, nonsmokers, etc.) is low, and if there is reason to believe that the property characterizing that category is an effect modifier (the effect of the exposure is different than among other categories), it is prudent not to include such individuals in the study base. Their inclusion could lead to the false impression that the results of the study would apply also to these categories, although their number was too small for any conclusions at all. Even if critical readers would not walk into this trap, investigating categories devoid of information means a waste of money and efforts for the investigator.

Because an "exposed" cohort is defined as having a certain exposure, only *effects caused by one exposure,* namely that particular exposure, can be studied at a time. For example, if the exposure of interest is silica dust, it is not feasible to study the effects of other dusts, say asbestos, in the same setting. However, sometimes it may be possible to form subcohorts with different combinations of exposures, provided the material is large enough and the exposure data are sufficiently detailed and accurate. On the other hand, the cohort design permits the study of *several diseases at a time*. Hence, one can study both the overall and cause-specific mortality from the same cohort. Provided measurements of other morbidity indicators exist or can be organized, one can also study different manifestations of the same disease. If the data are historical, morbidity measurements that can be used for the purpose of scientific research rarely exist, because softer indicators of morbidity than death have usually not been recorded in a systematic way. However, a prospective cohort study can well be designed to measure, for example, both coronary mortality and different severities of morbidity, such as nonfatal infarction, onset of electrocardiographic changes (e.g., S–T depressions at rest and after exercise), and symptoms of angina.

The occurrence relation between several diseases to one exposure can be investigated in a cohort-based census study at the same time.

Whenever a census approach has been taken, the tradition in occupational medicine has been to study a cohort base, not a dynamic population base. In a cohort, all members who have been enrolled stay in the cohort forever, even after they have *incurred the disease or died*. Consequently, all those who were originally exposed must be traced, and their outcome must be registered; the fact that their exposure has ceased does not influence their cohort membership. Operationally, a cohort study will, of course, end some day, but conceptually the cohort members remain in the cohort forever (Figure 2).

Cohorts are of two types, depending on how they have been designed. In the first type, all those who have been exposed at a certain point in time are enrolled (cross-sectional cohort base). In the second, those who have entered the exposure during a certain period of time are enrolled (entry cohort base). There are important differences between these two approaches.

With a cross-sectional cohort-base design, self-selection may have occurred before the formation of the cohort; those who were still exposed when the cohort was defined may be healthier than those who had quit employment after a short period of exposure. With the entry-base design, new workers are accepted during a certain time period. This inclusion of new workers, in turn, leads to a high proportion of cohort members who are designated to remain in the exposed category for a short time only. Because turnover is

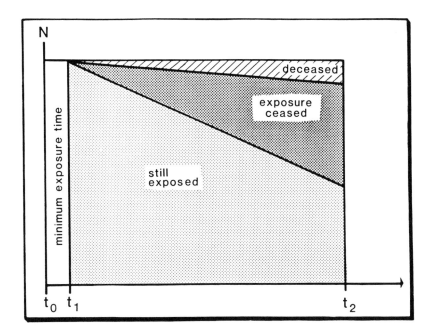

Figure 2. Composition of a cohort during follow-up. The cohort ages during that time.

always highest at the beginning of employment, the result is short exposure times for a large proportion of the cohort members. Moreover, those who tend to quit employment early may be socially different from those who are more stable.

If the population is large enough, one can focus the study on those who have remained exposed for some period of time by setting a minimum duration of exposure as one of the eligibility criteria. Especially when skilled occupations are being studied, many workers entering the cohort may have had similar exposure earlier, when employed by another company in the same branch of industry. Accounting for such exposure is important, although it requires additional work, because it makes the study more efficient by increasing the proportion of workers with longer exposure times.

However, in practice many cohort studies are hybrids of these two types. For example, the cohort may first be defined as a cross-sectional cohort base, comprising all those employed at a certain point in time, whereafter new entries are admitted during a period of time. Such a hybrid design complicates the interpretation of the results, but must often be used to achieve a large enough study material.

A cohort study can be either *retrospective* (historical) or *prospective*. In both instances the scientific structure is the same. A census of exposed individuals is defined at some point or period in time and followed thereafter, and the outcome is measured for all individuals. The difference is only in the timing. If the design is retrospective, the outcome has already occurred; if it is prospective, one has to wait for it.

A retrospective cohort is defined at some point in time or during some period in the past, say, 20 to 30 years earlier. The morbidity is then followed to the present, or for practical reasons, until 1 or $\frac{1}{2}$ year earlier so that the outcome data have become registered. (The registration delay is usually 2 to 4 months; it may vary from one country to another.) Tracing those who have quit their employment is important. One should try to find them all. In practice, such coverage cannot always be achieved. In the Nordic countries one can usually trace 97 to 99% of the subjects, but the result may be less successful in countries with weaker population registers. Failure to locate people usually depends either on the fact that the personal data, usually the personal identification number, have been wrong or on the fact that the person in question has turned asocial, having no address.

Successful tracing of all individuals should be the goal in cohort studies.

Whenever the proportion of untraceable cohort members is large, say, more than 5%, the question arises of whether or not the missing persons have the same vital status as those found by the tracing procedure. Marked differences would distort any conclusions based on the outcome of those who could be traced because persons who cannot be traced usually differ from the ones who can.

There are different ways of handling such missing data in the analyses. One is to dismiss missing persons completely by classifying them as "unknown." However, this procedure would mean loss of information because, after all, these individuals accrued some person-years of follow-up before they disappeared. Assuming the same mortality for them as for those with known vital status would imply that the missing persons did not differ from those found—a highly doubtful assumption. Another approach would be to consider them all alive, but then there would be an underestimation of the true effect of the exposure. Considering them all dead would, by the same token, overestimate this effect. The most recommendable method is to continue counting person-years until the last date the subject was known to be alive and to make no assumptions of vital status thereafter. Sometimes a cohort member is known to be dead, but the cause of death is unknown, either due to completely missing information or to inadequate data in the death certificate. One can either classify the causes of death for these individuals as "unknown" or, alternatively, assume the same distribution of deaths for the unknown as for the known cohort members. Again, the latter alternative assumes that there are no differences between these categories. Therefore it is better to classify the causes of death as "unknown."

Table 1. Layout of a Table Showing the Results of Cohort Data with Count Denominators

| Components of | Exposure Category | |
Disease Rate	Exposed	Unexposed
Cases	c_1	c_0
All subjects	N_1	N_0

Retrospective cohort studies are usually mortality studies because other indicators of morbidity are rarely available in register form. However, in some countries the cancer registers collect data on incident cancer cases, and therefore retrospective cancer incidence studies are possible. Data on permanent disability and long-term morbidity may also be available in some countries (e.g., in Finland from 1969 in a computerized form). However, changes in welfare legislation over time may render the interpretation of such data difficult.

A *prospective cohort* is defined as of the present and then followed into the future. By a prospective design one can also study morbidity indicators other than death. Exposure measurements can be made regularly and systematically, which is a great advantage over a retrospective design. The follow-up of those who quit their employment can also be planned more effectively. Otherwise, the design of a prospective cohort does not differ much from that of a retrospective study.

Table 1 shows the principles of tabulating data from a cohort study employing an ad hoc reference cohort. In this example, the exposed and the reference cohorts are compared with respect to one disease only.

The proportion of diseased in the exposed cohort is $R_1 = c_1/N_1$ and that of the reference cohort $R_0 = c_0/N_0$. Then $RR = R_1/R_0$.

Example 6. Suppose that a 5-year follow-up of 343 viscose rayon workers and 343 workers of a paper mill shows that 14 viscose workers but only 3 paper workers have died of myocardial infarction. Substituting the letters in Table 1 with these figures would give the following result:

| Components of | Exposure Category | |
Disease Rates	Viscose workers	Paper workers
Cases	14	3
All subjects	343	343

$$\widehat{RR} = \frac{14/343}{3/343} = 4.7$$

As already stated in Chapter 2, when the RR is greater than 1, the morbidity of the exposed cohort is higher than that of the reference cohort. In this example, there indeed was a reference cohort, but often the total and cause-specific mortality of the exposed cohort is compared to expected figures derived from the general population, adjusted for age, gender, and calendar time, to yield the SMR instead of the standardized RR. An SMR in excess of 100 suggests an increased mortality among the exposed. If, on the other hand, the SMR is below 100, the interpretation is not straightforward because the so-called healthy worker effect often confounds the comparison (see Chapter 5).

Table 2. Complementary Information from RR and RD[a]

Disease	O	E	RR	RD (per 10,000)
Common	150	100	1.5	50
Rare	2	0.01	200	1.99

[a] The observed (O) and expected (E) numbers are given as numerators of incidence rates/10,000 person-years.

The RR and the SMR are computed as point estimates ("best guesses"). Because any point estimate varies randomly, a confidence interval should always be computed for these ratios (see Chapter 2).

The RR and the SMR describe the magnitude of the risk — the *strength of the effect* of the exposure. The importance of the problem in terms of public health, that is, how *many* additional cases of the disease in question are caused by the exposure, is better described by the rate difference (RD) estimated as

$$\widehat{RD} = \frac{c_1}{N_1} - \frac{c_0}{N_0}$$

Table 2 compares the information provided by the $\widehat{RR}$ and $\widehat{RD}$ in a hypothetical example of two studies of rare and common diseases. When the disease is rare, even a very high $\widehat{RR}$ may be connected with a low $\widehat{RD}$ (only a few additional cases). By contrast, if the disease is common, a rather low $\widehat{RR}$ does not exclude the possibility of a relatively large $\widehat{RD}$ (many additional cases). One should, therefore, regard both measures when analyzing the results of a cohort study.

As already stated, retrospective cohort studies are usually mortality studies using the mortality experience of the general population as the reference. In Example 7 such a retrospective cohort study is illustrated.

Example 7. Coggon et al.[3] studied the mortality of workers exposed to styrene in the manufacture of glass-reinforced plastics. The subjects were identified from the personnel and wage records of eight British companies. For each subject the name, gender, address, date of birth, national insurance number, and a history of the jobs held during the whole employment were recorded, including the dates of first and last employment. Altogether 8354 subjects were identified from the records, but data were incomplete for 405 of them. A further 205 subjects could not be found in the files of the registers available, and 175 subjects emigrated during the study period. For both of these groups the person-years were computed as long as they were employed by one of the companies. Because these subjects stayed in the study for at least some time, they were not completely excluded from the study and hence the population qualifying for analysis included all those who had complete initial records, or 7949 subjects, 6638 being men and 1311 women.

Each job held was then classified, with the help of the management and staff of the companies, according to the potential exposure to styrene. This identification was made before the investigators had any knowledge of the subjects' vital status, an important precaution against observer error (see Chapter 5). The exposure was classified into four categories according to intensity. No hygienic data were available until 1975, but from then on the styrene concentration had been measured in four of the factories. This is a very common situation in retrospective studies, and in such cases some estimate of the real exposure must be made on the basis of whatever data are available. The authors estimated, from the available measurements, that the high-exposure category corresponded to an 8-h time-weighted average exposure of 40 to 100 ppm. Personal respirators were not considered to have affected the exposure level to any significant degree. Of the other exposures that had occurred, glass fiber, acetone, methyl ethyl ketone, organic peroxides and, in two factories, asbestos, were considered to have been the most important.

Members of the cohort were traced through the British National Health Service's Central Register and National Insurance Index, and their vital status as of 31 December 1984 was determined. Death certificates for those who had died were obtained, and the causes of death were coded according to the ninth revision of the International Classification of Diseases. The mortality of the cohort was compared to that of the national population of England and Wales by the person-year method. The analyses included subgroupings according to length of employment and grade of potential exposure to styrene.

The cohort was first analyzed as a homogeneous population, with the exception of one plant, characterized by poorer than average records. The cause-specific mortality analysis of this full cohort did not reveal anything remarkable. None of the SMR values computed for any group of diseases or for different cancer sites were statistically significantly in excess of 100 (i.e., all the lower 95% confidence limits were below 100). Leaving the analysis at this point would not have been correct because only 2458 workers had been working exposed to styrene for more than 1 year. Moreover, 1376 subjects had been exposed to low intensities only (partly overlapping with the former category), and about a fourth of the workers had entered the exposure so recently that the latency period for work-related cancers would probably not have been long enough.

All these considerations tend to dilute an analysis of a cohort if it is treated as a homogeneous population. Therefore, the authors made subanalyses for cancer mortality by grade of exposure, length of exposure, time since first exposure, and calendar period of first exposure to styrene. None of these further analyses revealed any excess of cancer of any site, but such a subgrouping resulted in low expected numbers in each comparison. Hence a superficially large material, after all, proved to be substantially smaller when the analysis was directed toward those subcategories carrying the information. The point is that the number of individuals carrying information, namely, those exposed to high concentrations long ago and for a long period of time, was actually rather small. This is a very common problem in epidemiologic cancer studies.

The authors did not adjust for other concurrent (confounding) exposures in their analysis. Because the results of the study turned out to be negative, there was no reason to analyze the data for separated effects of various exposures, but, had the result been positive in any of the subsets, or for any type of tumor, further analysis of the role of potential causes other than styrene would have been necessary.

The study summarized in Example 7 is a typical example of a retrospective cohort study. Only mortality could be studied, there were some problems with securing accurate exposure data, and, although the number of subjects enrolled in the cohort was large, the number of those actually conveying information turned out to be comparatively small.

A prospective cohort study is a good alternative to a retrospective study whenever the outcome follows the exposure rather soon (short latency time) and whenever one wishes to study morbidity indicators other than death. Example 8 illustrates these points.

Example 8. Tola et al.[16] were interested in the sequence of appearance of the hematologic manifestations of lead toxicity. For this purpose they selected 33 workers who entered lead exposure for the first time in their lives. That no lead exposure indeed had occurred earlier was checked by a thorough occupational history and biochemical tests. A follow-up of these workers was then initiated and the concentrations of lead in the blood (B–Pb) and urine (U–Pb) served as exposure indicators, while the blood hemoglobin value, the hematocrit value, the activity of erythrocyte δ-aminolevulinic acid dehydratase (ALA-D), and the concentrations of δ-aminolevulinic acid (ALA) and coproporphyrin (CP) in the urine served as outcome parameters. The analytical methods were standardized and checked regularly by quality control programs. According to the study protocol, samples were taken before the start of exposure, at the second, fourth, and sixth day after it, and then at weekly intervals until the end of the third month. During the fourth month, two further samples were taken at 2-week intervals.

The advantages of the prospective design were obvious in this study. There was the opportunity to do repeated measurements of the morbidity indicators, the possibility of regularly monitoring the exposure, and the chance of using several "soft" outcome indicators at a time. In addition, an analytical quality control program improved the reliability of the various measurements. However, there were also problems. The planned sampling schedule did not work perfectly during weekends, sick leaves, and other days off work (e.g., after night shifts). Several cohort members quit their job rather early, and for two workers the B–Pb concentration exceeded the then hygienic standard of 70 μg/100 mL so that they had to be transferred to an unexposed job. Only 18 of the original 33 workers remained in the study until the end of the planned 4 months of follow-up.

The results showed that the ALA-D activity became inhibited as the B–Pb concentrations rose, without any time lag, whereas the excretion of CP and ALA increased only after 2 to 3 weeks. The relationship between the concentrations of urinary ALA and CP, on the one hand, and the B–Pb, on the other, were the same as reported in earlier cross-sectional studies. Although all the blood hemoglobin values remained within normal limits, a slight decrease could be shown during the 4-month follow-up. The advantage of the prospective design versus the more conventional cross-sectional design was that the time sequence for the various toxic effects of lead could be demonstrated.

Rapid turnover at the beginning of employment means loss of material when an entry cohort is being followed prospectively. Especially when baseline data are required (i.e., the subjects are examined before the start of employment), the turnover causes losses in terms of unnecessary work (from the point of view of the study) because those who quit the job early do not contribute any information. Later turnover is not as much of a problem for the study because such individuals have, after all, already accrued some exposure, and their results convey at least some information. However, tracing them may be laborious, and often they have lost their motivation to contribute to the study, meaning that they may refuse further examinations.

In the study summarized in Example 8 an ethical issue also arose. The researcher must never allow the exposure to reach dangerous levels. If there is such a tendency, the researcher must inform the worker and suggest a transfer to less exposed tasks to the employer. In practice then, the worker is lost from the study, especially if the exposure reaches dangerous levels early in the course of the follow-up.

When the point estimate of the RR is greater than 1, the share of the excess that is caused by the exposure in question, which has been called the attributable proportion[15] or the *etiologic fraction* (EF) among the exposed,[12] can be computed as follows:

$$\widehat{EF} = \frac{O/E - 1}{O/E} = \frac{RR - 1}{RR}$$

where O = the observed number of cases in the exposed cohort and
E = the expected number of cases or, alternatively, the number observed in the reference group of equal size.

Example 9. Suppose 30 cases of lung cancer are observed in a cohort of chromate workers. Let the expected number be 11. Then O/E = 30/11 = 2.8, and $\widehat{EF}$ = (2.8 − 1)/2.8 = 0.64. In other words, 64% of the cases (point estimate) can be ascribed to chromate exposure, of course, provided the study is valid.

The etiologic fraction found in a particular study cannot be generalized because it depends on the strength and duration of the exposure and on other properties of that specific exposed population. In addition, its interpretation is complex. Because it is a proportion, it is also influenced by the strength of other concomitantly occurring risk factors. If other risk factors decrease in strength, the etiologic fraction of the exposure in question automatically increases even if the level of exposure and the number of cases remain the same.[4] Finally, because the concepts of multifactorial etiology are complex, the interpretation of the meaning of the etiologic fraction becomes even more difficult (see Chapter 1). The effect of two different etiologic fractions may be additive or synergistic. If it is synergistic or multiplicative, the joint effect of the single factors exceeds their sum.

Example 10. The combined effect of smoking and exposure to asbestos on the incidence of lung cancer is a classic example of synergism. For example, in a study by Hammond et al.,[7] the RR for lung cancer among nonsmoking workers, not exposed to asbestos, was defined as 1. The point estimate of the RR for asbestos-exposed nonsmokers was 5.2 and that for smokers not exposed to asbestos was 10.9. However, the estimate of the RR for asbestos-exposed smokers was as high as 53.2, which is very close to 5.2 x 10.9. The figures concerned those lung cancer cases that appeared 20 years or more after the commencement of exposure. The authors estimated that 92% of the cases could have been prevented if smoking alone were eliminated, and 81% if asbestos exposure alone were eliminated among smoking asbestos workers. "Elimination" means the theoretical situation in which the workers would never have smoked, or would never have been exposed to asbestos. The effect of quitting smoking or leaving asbestos exposure at a later stage is not implied by this exercise. However, the figures show how strong the preventive effect can be if one of two multiplicative factors is "eliminated."

Case-Referent Sampling of the Cohort Base

During recent years it has become more and more common to collect information from a cohort-type study of base by sampling. A variant of this design has earlier been called a "nested case-referent design." In order for this type of design to be efficient, the cohort base should differ from the one designed for a census type of study, which concentrates on subjects with high and/or longstanding exposure. If a sampling approach — a case-referent sampling of the cohort base — is planned, the cohort base should include both heavily exposed, less exposed (in terms of either intensity or duration, or both), and unexposed individuals to ensure exposure contrasts. The design of the cohort base should apply experimental principles of exposure distribution exactly as was discussed earlier for census-type studies.

Case-referent studies based on dynamic populations are still more common than cohort-based case-referent designs. In many respects they are executed in the same way. Therefore, a more thorough description of their common features is given in the section "Dynamic Population-Based Studies," while this text concentrates on aspects that are typical of cohort-based case-referent studies.

All the cases occurring in a cohort base are gathered to form the case series, but only a random sample of the base is drawn to serve as the reference group. The investigators then gather information on the exposure by interviewing cases and referents or their close relatives, checking the employers' personnel rolls, or constructing a job-exposure matrix (JEM) (see Chapter 3). If the exposure of concern increases the morbidity, more cases than referents will be classified as "exposed," provided the exposure gradient is sufficiently large in the cohort base. It is indeed important to ensure, in the planning of the study, that the cohort base comprises a sufficient proportion of slightly exposed and even unexposed individuals, along the same lines of thinking as when an "exposed" cohort is being contrasted to an "unexposed" one in a census-based study. If one originally planned to have an "exposed" and a "reference" cohort, it is only natural to combine them.

A case-referent approach within a cohort comprising "exposed" subjects only is ineffective because the contrasts are too slight. This aspect must be particularly stressed because many studies nowadays start as conventional cohort studies (SMR studies) with emphasis on strong exposure of long duration and with the general population as the reference category. Later a case-referent analysis of the original, exposed cohort is thought of as a means to avoid the problems arising from the healthy worker effect (see Chapter 5) and enable the researcher to penetrate the exposure histories (of a sample of the cohort) better. However, such a constellation is inefficient (effect-masking) because there are, by design, no really unexposed individuals in the cohort base. Therefore the analysis of such a cohort base by a case-referent design does not yield the information desired. The solution is to form the cohort base in a different way from the very beginning. Unexposed individuals can be found from other workplaces with exposure patterns that differ from the ones providing the exposed population. One can also include different types of personnel employed by the same company in the cohort base.

The cases can either be matched with one or more referents from the study base, or the cases and referents can be left unmatched. Matching is currently becoming less and less popular because it can introduce negative confounding (see Chapter 5). Tables 3 and 4 (in the next section) show the layout for presenting the results of a case-referent comparison. The OR is an indirect estimate of the risk of disease among the exposed, relative to the unexposed. It is derived by comparing the exposure frequencies of the cases with those of a sample of the cohort base (or of noncases).

This type of case-referent study is, like all other studies, efficient only if enough cases of the disease of interest have occurred in the study base. "Enough" is, of course, a vague term; it can be taken to mean at least some 40 to 50 cases. Having that many cases may require a large cohort base, especially if the disease of interest is uncommon in the general population. However, because the exposure history will be penetrated only for a relatively small part of the study population, namely, the cases and the referents, the requirement of a large study base is not necessarily economically prohibitive.

A sampling of the cohort base is usually more cost-efficient than a conventional census-based cohort design.

In a conventional (census-based) cohort study, those who do not incur the disease under study contribute only by giving information to the denominator (person-years), and the effort devoted to gathering their exposure data (before the outcome is known) can be said to have been wasted. If the cohort base is sampled, all the relevant information can be gained from a comparison of the cases with a sample of the base. There is no need to gather data from the rest of the population, which usually amounts to 80 or 90% of the whole material.

As already mentioned, the cohort base can be designed to "enrich" the exposure if the study material is selected so that the proportion of exposed cases and referents becomes much higher. It should be noted, however, that the more common the disease in the study base, the more the estimate of the OR overestimates the true RR if the referents are noncases. A random sampling of the base to obtain referents, whereby cases can become referents in addition to being cases, overcomes this problem.

Example 11. Partanen et al.[14] designed a cohort base to investigate a possible connection between respiratory cancer and exposure to some chemicals used in the wood industry (formaldehyde, chlorophenols, some fungicides, etc.). In this example, only formaldehyde is considered, however. The study material was gathered from 19 hardboard, plywood, and formaldehyde glue plants and sawmills.

The cohort base was defined as the follow-up of men who were hired by these plants between 1944 and 1966 and had at least 1 year of employment. All in all, 7307 men complied with these criteria. Before the start of the study the researchers estimated that 28% of the individuals had been exposed to formaldehyde. Hence there were sufficient exposure contrasts in the study base.

All in all, 136 cases of respiratory cancer had occurred in the study base. An experienced pathologist went through all the cases by reviewing hospital and autopsy records and slides, if available. Three cases had an incorrect diagnosis and were removed from the case series, which comprised 133 cases after this exclusion. For each case, three referents were chosen (altogether 408) from among the same cohort base. They were matched according to year of birth. In addition, the referent was to be free of respiratory cancer and alive at the time of the diagnosis of the case. Otherwise the referents were selected randomly. The exposure histories of the cases and referents were gathered from the beginning of employment, and an experienced hygienist constructed a job-exposure matrix (JEM) on the basis of visits to each plant and the use of all the historical hygienic measurements available. In a few instances, he measured the present formaldehyde concentration when visiting the plant.

A JEM was constructed separately for each task in each plant and separately for different periods of calendar time. The hygienist was unaware of the case-referent status of the subjects. The data were collected from the employers' records and complemented by interviews of foremen. In addition, a question-naire was given each case and referent or their next-of-kin. The occupational histories were then coded into occupational classes according to the JEM. The occupational histories and the JEM were combined by a computer, and exposure indices for formaldehyde (and other) exposures were computed with allowance for latency periods of different length. Next, OR values were computed for different types of comparisons (without latency, with different latency periods, standardized for confounding exposures). The point estimates of the OR values ranged between 0.82 and 1.95, but, because none of them differed statistically from unity, the study gave no clear indications in favor of a relationship between exposure to formaldehyde and respiratory cancer. Neither could such a con-nection be ruled out because the study had a rather weak statistical power due to the small number of exposed cases and the comparatively short follow-up period for many of the workers.

As was evident from the example, the study base was the follow-up of a cohort which had been designed to include both exposed and unexposed individuals so that exposure contrasts could be ensured. The exposure fre-quency to formaldehyde was common enough (28%) to make the study ef-ficient in that sense. It was much more common than it would have been in a case-referent study based on the entire general population. The exposure was recorded for all the cases, but only for a sample of the referents, as is usually done in this type of study. The purpose of the sample of referents was to measure the exposure frequency in the study base and thereby provide an estimate of the incidence rate ratio. In hindsight one can see that, instead of a sample of noncases, a sample of the whole study base could alternatively have been taken. In this example, the small difference in incidence rates between the exposed and unexposed persons could have been due to chance, and therefore the study gave inconclusive results on the carcinogenicity of formaldehyde. How great the economic advantage is of studying only a sample of the referents can be shown by some figures. Instead of having to examine the work histories of all the 7307 cohort members, only those of 408 referents and 133 cases had to be collected—indeed an immense saving of effort.

It should also be pointed out that the case diagnoses were confirmed by a pathologist. In a cohort study, using the general population as the reference material for computing the SMR, checking the diagnoses of the exposed cases would have been incorrect because no such check of the diagnoses of the reference population would have been possible. However, in this example, no SMR values were (or could be) computed for the cohort. Instead, the issue was to compute an OR for the cancer risk among the exposed on the basis of the cohort experience alone, by comparing the numbers of exposed cases and referents. In such a constellation, it is important to verify that the cases indeed are cases. Otherwise a dilution of any true effect would ensue. In this example, the proportion of misdiagnoses turned out to be only 3 out of 60, or 5%, which would have been a marginal source of error only. However, often the proportion of misdiagnoses is higher.

Choosing referents from among those still alive when the case was diagnosed led to asymmetry of the vital status between the cases and the referents. Because the prognosis of respiratory cancer is poor, there were comparatively more referents than cases alive when the exposure histories were gathered. The subjects themselves usually give a more-detailed exposure history than a close relative, so there was a risk of information bias (see Chapter 5). In this study the overrepresentation of alive referents would conceivably have resulted in a negative (effect-masking) information bias. A scrutiny of the exposure histories showed that this assumption was correct indeed, and the bias was controlled by analyzing the data obtained from alive cases and referents separately from those obtained from close relatives.

DYNAMIC POPULATION-BASED STUDIES

A dynamic population (Figure 3) differs from a cohort in the sense that it has a turnover of individuals. New people enter the population in the course of the follow-up period, while others move out of it.

Because tracing cohort members who have left employment can be difficult, a dynamic population base may, when superficially regarded, seem more cost-effective than a cohort base in census-type studies. Indeed, in the realm of public health, dynamic population bases are often preferred over cohort bases. However, as pointed out earlier, this approach is not without problems when work-related diseases are being studied. In order to overcome the distortions caused by outcome-selective turnover (e.g., sick persons quit the "exposed" job), a dynamic population must be so large that those changing employment would still remain in it. A census of such a large population would seldom be feasible. The other option is, of course, a design based on sampling.

Principles of Case-Referent Design

A sampling design of a dynamic population base is identical to the classic case-referent (case-control) design. All the cases that have occurred are gathered from the study base, and are contrasted to a sample of referents drawn from the same base. This sample has traditionally been a sample of noncases, but recently Miettinen[12] and others have advocated for drawing the sample from the whole base. This practice can result in a case being included among the referents in addition to being a case.

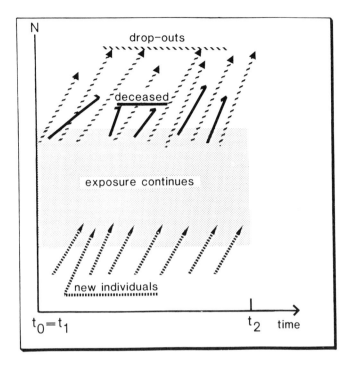

Figure 3. Structure of a dynamic population. There is a turnover of individuals, and, if the turnover is balanced, a dynamic population does not age during the follow-up.

Conceptually there is no difference between a case-referent and a census design. In both instances, the issue is to study whether a certain exposure causes a certain disease. The difference lies only in the method by which the information is gathered. One studies all the members of the base in a census approach, as against all the cases, but only a sample of referents in a case-referent approach. Although these two study types are different at the empirical level, conceptually they are not.

When the cases have been identified, a sample is drawn from the study base (or from noncases) to form the reference group, and the exposure histories of the cases and referents are gathered for the analysis. An indirect measure of the exposed individuals' risk to incur the disease in question (in relation to the risk of the unexposed) can then be obtained from the differences in the exposure frequencies. Exposed and unexposed cases provide the numerators of the estimated incidence rates. Information on the denominators derives from the exposed and unexposed referents (see Table 3).

Figure 4 shows the design of a case-referent study. It is important that the case diagnosis is correct because nondifferential misdiagnoses mask a true effect of the exposure. Therefore, to verify the diagnosis, one should check all available sources of information, such as hospital and autopsy records.

CASE–REFERENT STUDY

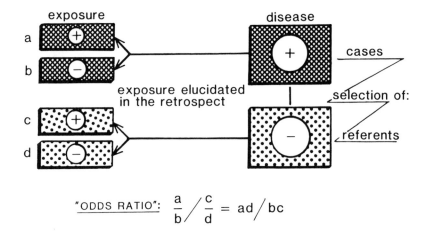

$$\text{"ODDS RATIO":} \quad \frac{a}{b} \Big/ \frac{c}{d} = ad \Big/ bc$$

Figure 4. Layout of a case-referent study.

The cases can be selected from national or local registers of causes of death, from a cancer register, from hospitals, and from many other sources, provided the diagnostic accuracy is good. Many registers do not fulfill the criteria for valid sources of cases. In cancer studies, it may even be important to specify the histological type of the tumor because different types may have different etiologies. An experienced pathologist as a member of the research team can do much to improve the diagnostic accuracy. If the accuracy is poor, and if it cannot be improved, abandoning the project may be the best solution.

In a case-referent study, the exposure histories of cases and referents are compared. The cases provide the numerators of the estimated incidence rates. Information for the denominators derives from the referents.

The referents can be selected in many ways, but they must belong to the same study base as the cases. Because a case-referent study is often based on interviews or questionnaires, that is, anamnestic data, it is important to ensure full cooperation of the referents. While a sick person (the case) usually sees some rationale in an interview, healthy persons may hesitate to answer a long questionnaire or respond in an interview whose relevance may not be obvious to them. Even those who cooperate may not give a history that is as detailed and accurate as those of the cases (see Chapter 5). For this reason, many researchers prefer to use patients with another disease as referents. Again, such referents should belong to the same study base as the cases. They should, therefore, be selected from the same hospital. This hospital should be the one they would have attended, had they had the case disease. The same rule applies for other sources of information, for example, registers.

Many ethical aspects should be considered when sick persons, and also close relatives to deceased persons, are interviewed. Therefore the interviewer must be considerate and empathetic, and the interview can only be done with the full consent of the subject (see Chapter 8).

Because the case-referent design relies on the exposure information obtained in interviews of patients with a certain disease—the particular disease under study—along with a sample of the study base, the referents, the connection with harmful exposures can be investigated for only one disease at a time in a particular study. By contrast, this design allows the concomitant study of the effect of several different exposures. This approach is often used in so-called explorative studies having no prior hypothesis. However, the same study base can be utilized for several concomitant case-referent studies on different diseases, if feasible. For example, it may be practical to draw several case series of different tumors from a cancer register along with the same set of referents and to mail the questionnaires simultaneously. If so, one is dealing with several case-referent studies utilizing the same study base (e.g., the experience of the dynamic population of the whole country during 3 years).

Because of the anamnestic nature of the exposure data, great care must be taken to ensure that the quality of the information is symmetric. These problems are further discussed in Chapter 5.

A case-referent study can investigate the occurrence relation between one disease and several exposures simultaneously.

The cases and the referents can be sampled and analyzed either as *independent series* or as *matched groups*. One referent can be matched to each case; the design is then a *matched-pair design*. If two referents are matched to each case, one speaks about *triplets*. Sometimes three or even four referents are matched to one case. Provided the costs of studying more referents, matched or unmatched, are not prohibitive, a greater number of referents improves the stability of the estimate of the OR and thereby makes the study more size efficient. However, in general, the gains of having more than four referents for each case are marginal.

Unmatched Case-Referent Studies

Table 3 shows the principles of comparing data from an unmatched case-

Table 3. Layout of a Table Showing the Results of an Unmatched Case-Referent Study

	Exposure Classification		
	Exposed	**Unexposed**	**Total**
Cases	c_1	c_0	$c_1 + c_0 = c$
Base sample	n_1	n_0	$n_1 + n_0 = n$
Total subjects	$c_1 + n_1$	$c_0 + n_0$	$c + n$

referent study. One exposure frequency is compared at a time, and similar tables can be constructed for each exposure under study. From this constellation, the odds of exposure among the cases, and the odds of exposure among the referents, can be computed and divided to yield the exposure odds ratio, OR. For the cases, the exposure odds is c_1/n_1, and for the referents it is c_0/n_0. The estimate of the OR is then:

$$\widehat{OR} = \frac{c_1/n_1}{c_0/n_0} = \frac{c_1 n_0}{c_0 n_1}$$

The OR is an indirect measure of the risk for the exposed to incur the disease, as compared with the corresponding risk of the referents. If more cases than referents have been exposed, the OR is in excess of 1, and, conversely, if the referents have been more frequently exposed, the OR is below 1. The OR is not exactly the same measure as the RR of a cohort study but, given certain conditions, the RR can be approximated from the OR. First, there must not be selection bias (see Chapter 5), that is, both the cases and the referents must be representative of the base population. Second, the disease must be rare in the study base (rare is a vague concept, but below 5% can be considered "rare"). However, under certain conditions, the RR corresponds to the OR even without a rare disease assumption.[1,6,11]

> *Example 12.* Suppose we are interested in the connection between chronic bronchitis and occupational dust exposure from a series of patients coming to the health center of a large company with a broad range of different exposures. Suppose also that the criteria for chronic bronchitis are agreed upon. The next patient seeking medical advice could be the referent. Suppose that the study comprises 100 cases of chronic bronchitis and 100 referents. Let 40 cases and 15 referents be exposed to dust (according to preset criteria). Then $c_1 = 40$, $c_0 = 60$, $n_1 = 15$, and $n_0 = 85$. Consequently,
>
> $$\widehat{OR} = \frac{40 \times 85}{60 \times 15} = 3.78$$

Matched Case-Referent Studies

Often the referents are matched to the cases with regard to potential confounders, such as age, gender, and area of residence (see Chapter 5). The

Table 4. Layout of a Table Showing Results of Matched Case-Referent Study (One-to-One Matching)

Cases	Referents	
	Exposure (+)	Exposure (−)
Exposure (+)	f_{++} [a]	f_{+-}
Exposure (−)	f_{-+}	f_{--}

[a] "f" stands for frequency of pairs.

procedure is to select one or more referents for each case on the basis of these matching criteria (e.g., age within 3 years, same gender, same municipality or same type of district of habitation, namely, urban or rural, same smoking category). The more properties used for matching, the more difficult to find referents.

The number of referents to be selected for each case depends to a great extent on the availability of cases and referents. If there are few available cases, for example, if the disease is rare in the study base, one can increase the statistical power of the study by drawing multiple referents for each case.[10] However, if the limiting factor is economic, or if the problem is to find enough interviewers, which may also be due to reasons other than economic ones, using too much of one's restricted funds to interview a large number of referents is not always worthwhile. A one-to-one design may then be optimal. The same is true if the availability of referents is restricted in relation to the availability of cases.

The analysis of a matched series focuses on the discordant pairs, namely, those in which either the case or the referent has been exposed, but not the other pair member. Concordant pairs (both the case and the referent have been exposed or neither the case nor the referent has been exposed) are not included in the analysis. Table 3 shows the presentation of the results from a matched-pair series (one-to-one matching). The analysis does not involve the numbers in f_{++} and f_{--}; the ratio f_{+-}/f_{-+} carries all the information. Note that the letters denote pairs in Table 4, not individuals as in Table 3.

Example 13. The connection between nasal and sinonasal adenocarcinoma (NSNC) and previous exposure both to hardwood and softwood dust was investigated in a joint Nordic case-referent study.[9] All in all, 167 alive cases were interviewed by telephone. For each case a referent was selected and matched for age, gender, and country of residence. In the actual study two cases and one referent had been exposed only to hardwood dust; they have been omitted from this example for the sake of simplification. The number of pairs is therefore reduced from 167 to 164. Those who had been exposed to softwood only have been classified as unexposed in this example.

In one of the 164 pairs, both the case and the referent had been exposed to hardwood dust, f_{++} in Table 4. In 150 pairs out of 164, neither the case nor the referent had been exposed, f_{--} in Table 4. The interesting numbers are in f_{+-} and f_{-+}. The case, but not the referent, had been exposed in 12 pairs, hence, $f_{+-} = 12/164$. The referent but not the case had been exposed in one pair; consequently $f_{-+} = 1/164$. When these numbers are placed into Table 4, the constellation shown in Table 5 emerges.

Table 5. The Nordic Study on Nasal and Sinonasal Cancer[a]

	Referents	
Cases	**Exposure (+)**	**Exposure (−)**
Exposure (+)	1	12
Exposure (−)	1	150

[a] Some figures for exposure to wood dusts. The numbers denote pairs, not individuals.

The whole information of this study is in the ratio f_{+-}/f_{-+} which is $12/1 = 12$. The numbers in f_{++} and f_{--} are not used for the computation of the $\widehat{OR}$. The $\widehat{OR}$ of 12 is a point estimate; the CI_{95} is 2.4--59.2. Because the lower boundary is in excess of 1, the OR = 12 is statistically significant at the 5% level. In other words, the study confirmed the carcinogenicity of hardwood dust. Several other exposures were also investigated in that study, but this example suffices to illustrate the matched-pair design.

Had the pairs been broken and the material treated as an unmatched series, the result would have been as follows (note that the symbols are now from Table 3):

$$c_1 = 1 + 12 = 13$$
$$n_1 = 1 + 150 = 151$$
$$c_0 = 1 + 1 = 2$$
$$n_0 = 12 + 150 = 162$$

Those two cases and one referent who had been exposed to hardwood dust only, are still omitted. Now the concordant pairs are also included in the analysis and added to the cases and referents, respectively

$$\widehat{OR} = c_1 \times n_0/(n_1 \times c_0) = 13 \times 162/(151 \times 2) = 7$$

The matched analysis was more powerful in this example, but both approaches gave results of a similar type.

PROPORTIONATE MORTALITY STUDIES

Proportionate mortality studies have already been described in Chapter 2. In this context only a variant, the morbidity odds ratio (MOR) approach will be presented to illustrate the conceptual similarity between case-referent studies and this type of proportionate mortality studies. If a proportionate mortality study is done so that the exposure histories of patients having died from the disease under study are compared to those of patients having died from another disease (see Chapter 2), instead of in the conventional way, the study can be regarded as a special type of a case-referent study. The cause of death of interest, say, coronary heart disease, forms the case series. The reference causes can either be all other causes of death or some specific other cause of death that is neither caused nor prevented by the exposure under study. If one, instead of taking the ratio of the proportions of cause of death [the ratio of the proportions of the "case" cause to all causes of death in two populations, or $c_1/(c_1 + n_1)$ to $c_0/(c_0 + n_0)$, which yields the PMR, symbols as in Chapter 2], computes the ratio of the odds of of cases and referents being exposed (the ratio of the exposed/unexposed cases to the exposed/unexposed referent diagnoses), the resulting $\widehat{MOR}$ is:

$$\widehat{MOR} = \frac{c_1/n_1}{c_0/n_0} = \frac{c_1 n_0}{c_0 n_1}$$

The ratio $c_1 n_0/c_0 n_1$ is the same as the crude estimate of the OR, which shows the similarity of an MOR study to a true case-referent study (see Chapter 2). However, as long as the reference category is the general population, as is usually the case in PMR studies, the validity of the study does not reach that of a well-planned case-referent study of the conventional type.

INTERVENTION STUDIES

An intervention study differs from other epidemiologic study types in the sense that the investigator actively changes the exposure conditions. Alternatively, the effects of changes of the exposure conditions, brought about by other causes, can be studied. In this respect an intervention study bears some resemblance to an experiment. In fact, interventive epidemiology is often called experimental epidemiology.

Experimental epidemiologic studies can be subdivided into field trials, community intervention trials, and randomized clinical trials. (See, for example, Reference 15.) Very few intervention studies have been published from the field of occupational epidemiology.

In a *field trial,* the population is initially made up of individuals who are healthy with respect to the disease(s) under study. In general, the incidence of most diseases is low. Hence, large populations are needed for field trials, and they are therefore expensive. In the occupational setting, an example of a field trial could be the study of the preventive effect of the introduction of respirators on the incidence of some toxic manifestations of a certain chemical agent among exposed workers. Another could be the study of the preventive effects of a fitness program on low-back disorders among industrial workers.

A system for the continuous collection of data must be set up in all field trials, for example, periodic examinations of the subjects, regular registration of cases of illness, and a system for registering the reasons for dropout, whereby dropouts can be traced easily. Large workplaces having good occupational health care services usually offer better opportunities for securing such data than the public health setting. The process of intervention in field trials must ensure good comparability of the study groups. Care must also be taken to minimize the information bias that could arise from the researchers' observations of the morbidity. Blinding of the researchers is rarely feasible in occupational epidemiology. The same can be said of a random assignment scheme. Therefore, other methods of securing validity must be tried (see Chapter 5).

In a *community intervention trial,* the intervention takes place on a community-wide, not an individual, basis. In occupational epidemiology, an example of such an intervention trial would be the change in a plant from one method of production to another, whereby either the use of some toxic agent either ceases or, alternatively, some new chemical is being introduced.

A *randomized clinical trial* is an experiment with patients as subjects, and it is usually initiated to test a new treatment. This is the only type of interventive epidemiology that fulfills the criteria of a true experiment. A clinical trial can be defined as an experimental study in which the subjects (patients) are randomly assigned to a group which receives the new treatment or one which receives a placebo or some other treatment. The results of the different treatments are then compared. It is not ethically acceptable to use a placebo if an effective treatment is available. In such cases, the control patients usually receive a conventional treatment, and the efficacy of the new treatment is compared to that of the conventional one. In a clinical trial, the researcher is usually *blinded,* meaning that the treatments are coded, and the researcher unaware of which patients receive the new and which the old treatment. Blinding is one of the methods for controlling information bias (see Chapter 5). The patients are usually also blinded for the same reason; if so, the trial is said to be *double-blind.* Because of its pure experimental design, a randomized clinical trial should perhaps not be referred to as belonging to the realm of epidemiology. Randomized clinical trials are not done in occupational epidemiology, but provide a paradigm for nonexperimental studies in general (see Chapter 5).

With the exception of randomized clinical trials, intervention studies differ from true experiments because randomization is hardly ever possible. Furthermore, the control of concomitant other exposures is usually not feasible. Therefore many occupational intervention studies can, in a way, be regarded as extensions of cohort studies in which before–after comparisons are made in a quasiexperimental way. For ethical reasons, the exposure levels can only be lowered deliberately, not increased. However, sometimes ''natural'' circumstances, for example, the introduction of new production processes or methods, may cause the exposure level to increase. With good luck and a good portion of alertness, the epidemiologist can then use this constellation for an ''intervention'' study. Plant physicians have especially good opportunities for this type of study. It is less likely for an outsider to obtain access to such a situation.

Although intervention studies bear some resemblance to experiments, the impossibility to randomize the study material is a fundamental difference, at least in the occupational health setting.

If an intervention study is designed as the continuation of a cohort study, the baseline data have already been gathered during the first stage. After the intervention, the follow-up continues and the data are recorded in a similar way. Because many uncontrollable events, apart from the intervention, may confound the before–after comparison, it is recommended to enroll a reference cohort into the study. This reference cohort could either be unexposed, perhaps the original reference cohort used for the first stage of the study, or it could be a part of the exposed cohort, for which no intervention has been made, or both.

In an intervention study, before–after comparisons are made within the exposed cohort; in addition, comparisons should be made with a reference group.

Positive results of intervention studies are usually considered strong arguments in favor of the causality of an observed association, even in spite of the fact that intervention studies rarely reach the same degree of validity as experiments (see Chapter 9).

As already mentioned, intervention studies have been rare in the occupational health setting. Some interventive studies belonging to the realm of public health, but carried out in large workplaces (e.g., antismoking trials and other trials aimed at the reduction of coronary risk), are perhaps exceptions to this rule. The problem is that the epidemiologist can rarely influence the work conditions in such a systematic way that a valid study can be designed. Close collaboration with active and skilled plant physicians is the best way for academic researchers to achieve good results in interventive endeavors in industry.

In spite of good planning, an intervention study may face insurmountable logistic problems. For example, baseline data on morbidity may be lacking, the intervention, that is, the change in the work conditions, may result in selective turnover to other jobs (e.g., if the old process is substituted by very modern technology). The mere fact that something is changed may result in changes in health behavior or in the proneness to complain of symptoms (the so-called Hawthorne effect), before–after observations may not be comparable, a valid reference group cannot be found, and so forth. Diseases that have a long latency period (e.g., cancer) and have been induced long before the intervention often become manifest after the intervention, so it may be impossible to define when the effects of the intervention really become detectable. In any case, decades are required. Thus the long waiting period may render the study impractical or even irrelevant for practical purposes, such as prevention.

As already stated, if a reduction in the exposure reduces the occurrence of the diseases of interest, the causality of the association is supported (see Chapter 9). In addition, such a result has a particularistic (bound to time and place) significance if the morbidity of the target population has indeed been reduced. The proportion of the reduction of the morbidity that can be ascribed to the reduction of the exposure, the preventive fraction (PF) among the exposed, can be computed as follows:

$$PF = 1 - 0/E = 1 - RR$$

where 0 = the observed number of cases after the intervention,
E = the expected number of cases, had there been no intervention.

Example 14. The third stage of the Finnish carbon disulfide (CS_2) study can be regarded as a kind of intervention.[13] The objective of the study was to investigate whether exposure to CS_2 was a true risk factor for coronary heart disease. The study began in 1967 as a cross section of the study base; also, the proportionate mortality was investigated in retrospect. The next step was to form two cohorts, one comprising exposed and the other unexposed workers, and to follow their morbidity in coronary heart disease. The exposed cohort comprised 343 male workers who had been exposed to CS_2 for 5 years or more between 1942 and 1967 and who were alive in 1967. The concentration of CS_2 in the air had been measured occasionally since the 1940s and regularly since the 1950s. The exposure levels had been very high in the 1940s, about 60 to 120 mg/m³ in the 1950s, and 30 to 90 mg/m³ in the 1960s. The hygienic standard was 60 mg/m³ until 1975, when it was reduced to 30 mg/m³. The reference cohort was formed from 343 men employed by a nearby paper mill. How comparability was achieved is explained in Chapter 5.

During the first 5 years of prospective follow-up, 14 exposed and 3 unexposed men died of coronary heart disease. The point estimate of the RR was 4.67 with a CI_{95} of 1.35 to 16.1. Because the lower confidence limit was above 1 at the 5% level, the result was statistically significant. The significance of the result was also tested by a χ^2 test; the χ^2 value was 7.12, corresponding to a two-sided p = 0.0076.

These alarming results prompted the viscose company to take strong preventive actions. The measures can be regarded as epidemiologic intervention. The intervention comprised more effective ventilation, further encapsulation of the process, and stricter adherence to hygienic principles (e.g., enforced use of fresh air masks). As a result, the average CS_2 concentration dropped to half the levels before the intervention. All the workers who were considered under high risk of coronary heart disease, irrespective of why (high serum cholesterol level, elevated blood pressure, symptoms of angina, and electrocardiographic findings suggestive of coronary heart disease), were removed from exposure and placed in unexposed jobs. After these actions, only 17% of the originally exposed workers remained exposed. The year 1975 was considered the time when the intervention was completed, and, from that year on, the follow-up continued as a quasiintervention study. During the period 1975 to 1982, the coronary mortality fell to the same level as in the reference cohort (RR = 1.0). Thus both the before–after comparison and the comparison to the reference cohort showed that the intervention had indeed had preventive effects. The results of the intervention gave more credibility to the conclusion that CS_2 exposure is a risk factor for the development of coronary heart disease.

The preventive effect of the intervention can be computed as follows: Between July 1967 and the end of 1975, 19 exposed and 6 reference subjects died from coronary heart disease $(\widehat{RR} = 3.2)$. During the next 7 years, 19 men died in each cohort $(\widehat{RR} = 1)$. If we suppose that the mortality of coronary heart disease among the exposed had continued unchanged relative to the unexposed, 59 men would have died (E = 59). Since only 19 deaths from coronary heart disease occurred, the $\widehat{PF} = 1 - 19/59 = 68\%$.

This example illustrates some of the practical problems of intervention studies in the field of occupational epidemiology. First, the intervention did not happen momentaneously; it was a gradual process encompassing 2 to 3 years. Thus it is hard to tell exactly when the investigation changed from a cohort study to an intervention study. Second, the intervention was strongest for those whose exposure ceased completely, because they were transferred to unexposed jobs. However, the coronary risk of these men was initially higher than the average, the presence of a high level of coronary risk factors being the reason for transfer. Therefore, those who remained exposed were not comparable to those whose exposure ceased completely.

Although this study did not meet the criteria for a scientifically correctly performed intervention, it helped establish the causality of the connection between CS_2 exposure and coronary heart disease. At the practical level, it showed how fruitful close collaboration can be between occupational epidemiologists, on the one hand, and employers and workers, on the other. The researchers had good support from both parties during the entire course of the study, and that support was decisive for its success.

CHOICE OF STUDY DESIGN

In principle, no one type of study is superior to the others. The choice of study type therefore depends on a number of factors related to feasibility, efficiency, and validity. Practical considerations are more important than researchers, especially nonepidemiologists, usually appreciate. The same scientifically "true" result can, in principle, be achieved in more than one way, but often practical matters, such as availability of study material, funds, and manpower, decide which design is optimal under the prevailing circumstances. However, the general principle is that a longitudinal design is preferable to a cross-sectional one whenever the issue is to collect etiologic information. Cross-sectional designs can only study the prevalence of a disease. They are, in addition, prone to systematic errors. Because longitudinal studies are the main tools in etiologic epidemiology, the following discussion is restricted to the relative advantages and disadvantages of different longitudinal designs.

Prospective or Retrospective Timing

If the timing of the study is retrospective, both the exposure and the outcome have already occurred. Both retrospective cohort studies and case-referent studies, irrespective of the type of study base, share this property. The only time needed to obtain the results is the period it takes to plan the study, gather and analyze the data, and prepare the report. Although census studies of a cohort base may require some years, especially if the cohort is large and tracing dropouts is cumbersome, the whole procedure usually takes no more than 2 to 5 years. A case-referent sampling of the cohort base, utilizing cases that have already occurred, usually takes less time to complete. Although a couple of years may seem long to impatient health administrators, it is a short period in comparison with the time required for most prospective follow-up studies of cohort bases. Whenever knowing the scientific "truth" is urgent, for example, for regulative purposes, strong arguments speak in favor of a retrospective design.

However, retrospective designs also have their disadvantages. A difficult problem is that past exposure data are usually deficient or even lacking, as has been pointed out many times. Likewise, it is rare to find past reliable data on milder manifestations of morbidity, such as blood chemistry, functional tests, and diagnoses of minor diseases. Therefore, a retrospective cohort study must usually be restricted to the study of mortality. A case-referent study can be so planned that prevalent or incident new nonfatal manifestations of the disease in question are registered at a point in time or during a period of, say, 2 years, and the exposure histories of the cases and a sample of the referents are elucidated retrospectively. However, in this setting, as well as in all other studies dealing with nonfatal manifestations, the diagnosis must be straightforward and reliable.

The advantages of a prospective design are:

1. The study can be better planned than a retrospective study to comply with the researchers' needs
2. Exposure data can be collected systematically
3. Several different manifestations of a disease can be measured
4. Measurements and medical examinations can be repeated
5. The methods of measurement can be standardized and their validity can be checked

The greatest disadvantage of a prospective design is the time period required for obtaining the results. Chronic diseases often have a long latency period, perhaps spanning as many as 20 to 40 years. However, sometimes the waiting period is shorter, depending on the type of problem (see Example 8). An often heard claim is that the costs of prospective census-type studies are high. The matter is not quite that straightforward. Because a prospective census design allows the recording of many different morbidity indicators, not merely mortality, it is true that the total costs may rise considerably, and exceed those of a similar retrospective design by many times. However, if the prospective study utilizes the possibilities of collecting different types of morbidity data, it yields more information than a retrospective study, which is restricted to mortality. Therefore the *costs per unit of information* do not necessarily exceed those of a retrospective study, especially when the higher quality of the information (e.g., exposure data) is considered. If the prospective study only concerns mortality, the costs are not much different from those of a retrospective one. In order to reduce the costs of a prospective census-based follow-up of the cohort base, it is important to restrict the measurements to the most relevant morbidity indicators, and to avoid measuring the same conceptual entity through the use of too many empirical parameters. However, this recommendation for parsimony does not apply to exposure measurements, which, unfortunately, until very recently have been given too little emphasis in occupational epidemiology.

Census or Sampling

The specific hypothesis ''A causes B'' can, in principle, be tested either by a census design, whereby the presence of exposure is set as the inclusion criterion in the study base, or by a study of the cases of B and a sample of noncases with respect to past exposure. The subjects can either come from a cohort base or a dynamic population base. Both approaches are, in principle, equally correct for testing such a hypothesis. Hence validity and feasibility matters usually decide the choice of approach. That different approaches do lead to the same conclusion is illustrated by the history of searching for a connection between cigarette smoking and lung cancer. The first indication of this connection came from a case-referent study. It was found that relatively more lung cancer patients than referents had been smokers, a finding which indirectly indicated that smoking cigarettes increases the risk of incurring lung cancer. Later similar results were obtained from cohort studies. It was found that smokers got lung cancer much more often than nonsmokers. Finally, intervention studies showed that, after cessation of smoking, the risk of lung cancer dropped nearly to that of nonsmokers in about 10 years. In other words, the same result emerged irrespective of study type.

In practice, a case-referent design from a large study base is the only option if the disease is rare. Usually the most feasible study base is a follow-up of a large dynamic population, although, in principle, there is nothing preventing the use of a cohort base. However, for economic and other feasibility reasons it is difficult to form a cohort base large enough to provide a sufficient number of exposed cases. By the same token, whenever the exposure is rare in the general population, the most efficient study base is a follow-up of a cohort base, defined on the basis of the particular exposure. Having defined the cohort base, one can choose between a census or a classic cohort study or alternatively, a sampling of the study base or a case-referent study within the cohort base. The latter choice requires exposure contrasts within the study base, however. It is crucial to include as many subjects as possible who have or have had the particular rare exposure. Often this requires the enrollment of several companies and may, therefore, pose practical problems.

Common diseases can also be studied well with a dynamic population-based case-referent design. Likewise, common exposures can be studied by a cohort-base design.

A dynamic population-based case-referent design is the most efficient if the disease is rare. A census of a cohort base is the choice if the exposure is rare in the general population.

The greatest advantages of a case-referent over a census design are that the costs are lower and the input of manpower smaller. Most of the members of a study population do not incur the disease of interest. Nevertheless their exposure must be explored, and dropouts must be traced. This effort does not yield any real information. Only those subjects who incur the disease yield information. A case-referent sampling does not require such efforts.

If several hypotheses are combined, or if no prior hypothesis exists, there are no longer any options in study design. If the hypothesis is "exposure A causes diseases B_1, B_2, . . . B_i," or if the question is "what diseases are caused by A?," the only feasible epidemiologic design is that of a census study of a cohort base, formed on the basis of exposure to A. A census of a dynamic population base (e.g., of a plant) has not been a common design in occupational epidemiology because of the fear of bias caused by selective turnover of the work force.

If the hypothesis takes the form "disease B is caused by exposures A_1, A_2, . . . A_i," or if the question is "what are the causes of disease B?," a case-referent sampling design is the only epidemiologic option. Then the study groups are formed on the basis of the presence or absence of the disease B, and factors distinguishing cases from the rest of the base, represented by a sample, are being investigated. Such a study is usually carried out on a dynamic population, but alternatively the study base can be designed as a case-referent study within a cohort base, so designed that its members have had the opportunity for exposure to several different agents.

Example 15. Axelson et al.[2] designed a multiple case-referent study, the aim of which was to determine if exposure to arsenic compounds was connected with lung cancer, some other cancer forms, and CHD. In this example only lung cancer will be dealt with, however. The study base was a follow-up of the dynamic population living in some parishes around a large Swedish copper smelter. The cases were patients who had died of lung cancer, and the referents were people who had died of other causes, except for cancer or coronary heart disease. Both the cases and referents were drawn from local parish records. One of the problems with this study was that, according to the prior hypothesis, arsenic could not only cause lung cancer, but also some other diseases. Therefore, if persons who had died from such causes were to be included in the reference group, a true effect of arsenic exposure on lung cancer mortality would be masked. The researchers therefore formed separate case series for each suspected cause of death (e.g., lung cancer, some other cancers, CHD) and used those who had died of the remaining causes as the referents. One can regard this study as a conglomerate of case-referent studies, utilizing the morbidity experience of the same study base.

As always in retrospective studies, obtaining sufficiently good exposure data was a problem. The researchers requested an experienced safety engineer to classify the estimated exposure intensity for each case and each referent into the following three categories: (1) exposure clearly below the then hygienic standard of 0.5 mg/m^3, (2) exposure close to that level, and (3) exposure clearly in excess of that level (cf. Chapter 3).

Axelson and his co-workers allowed for a latency period in their data analysis. On the basis of the literature, they estimated the average latency period to be 34 to 36 years for arsenic-induced lung cancer. Therefore they decided to disregard exposures that had occurred during the 17 years preceding the diagnosis (half the estimated average latency time). This, of course, was an arbitrary decision. The results showed that the risk of contracting lung cancer was 4.6-fold (CI_{90} 2.2--9.6) for those exposed to arsenic, and there seemed to be an exposure–response relationship (nonsignificant) over the categories of exposure. In addition the point estimate of the RR of dying from coronary infarction was 2.2 (CI_{90} 1.2--3.5), which shows that the researchers were correct in not including this diagnosis in the reference category.

As stated before, a population-based case-referent design is inefficient if the exposure is rare in the study population. Exposure to arsenic is certainly rare in the Swedish general population. However, the researchers restricted the dynamic population base to encompass a few municipalities in the vicinity of the smelter. As a result, the exposure became common in the study base. Because of this "enrichment" the case-referent design could be applied effectively.

The choice of study design also depends on many circumstances other than those discussed in this chapter. Because these factors are related to validity aspects they are treated in Chapter 5. Both feasibility and validity aspects decide which approach is the best for the study of a scientific problem in a particular setting. Unfortunately these aspects may sometimes be conflicting. It is then up to the researcher to decide which of the options results in the most advantages and the least disadvantages.

REFERENCES

1. Axelson, O., "Elucidation of some epidemiologic principles," *Scand. J. Work Environ. Health* 9:231 (1983).
2. Axelson, O., E. Dahlgren, C. D. Jansson, and S. O. Renlund, "Arsenic exposure and mortality. A case referent study from a Swedish copper smelter," *Br. J. Ind. Med.* 35:8 (1978).
3. Coggon, D., C. Osmond, B. Pannett, S. Simmonds, P. Winter, and E. D. Acheson, "Mortality of workers exposed to styrene in the manufacture of glass-reinforced plastics," *Scand. J. Work Environ. Health* 13:94 (1987).
4. Cole, P. and F. Merletti, "Chemical agents and occupational cancer," *Environ. Pathol. Toxicol.* 3:399 (1980).
5. Fox, A. J. and A. M. Adelstein, "Occupational mortality: work or way of life?" *J. Epidemiol. Community Health* 32:73 (1978).
6. Greenland, S. and D. Thomas, "On the need for the rare disease assumption in case-control studies, *Am. J. Epidemiol.* 116:547 (1982).
7. Hammond, E.C., I. J. Selikoff, and H. Seidman, "Asbestos exposure, cigarette smoking and death rates," *Ann. N.Y. Acad. Sci.* 330:473 (1979).
8. Hernberg, S., T. Partanen, C.-H. Nordman, and P. Sumari, "Coronary heart disease among workers exposed to carbon disulphide," *Br. J. Ind. Med.* 27:313 (1970).
9. Hernberg, S., P. Westerholm, and K. Schultz-Larsen, et al. "Nasal and sinonasal cancer: connection with occupational exposure in Denmark, Finland and Sweden, *Scand. J. Work Environ. Health* 9:315 (1983).
10. Miettinen, O. S. "Individual matching with multiple controls in the case of an all-or-none response," *Biometrics* 25:339 (1969).
11. Miettinen, O. S. "Estimability and estimation in case-referent studies," *Am. J. Epidemiol.* 103:226 (1976).
12. Miettinen, O. S. *Theoretical Epidemiology: Principles of Occurrence Research in Medicine* (New York, John Wiley & Sons, 1985).
13. Nurminen, M. and S. Hernberg, "Effects of intervention on cardiovascular mortality among workers exposed to carbon disulphide: a 15-year follow-up," *Br. J. Ind. Med.* 42:32 (1985).
14. Partanen, T., T. Kauppinen, and M. Nurminen, et al. "Formaldehyde exposure and respiratory and related cancers: a case-referent study among Finnish woodworkers, *Scand. J. Work Environ. Health* 16:394 (1990).
15. Rothman, K. J. *Modern Epidemiology* (Boston, MA: Little, Brown, 1986).
16. Tola, S., S. Hernberg, and J. Nikkanen, "Parameters indicative of absorption and biological effect in new lead exposure: a prospective study, *Br. J. Ind. Med.* 30:134 (1973).

CHAPTER 5

Internal Validity, Precision, and Generalization

INTRODUCTION

The result of a specific study can either be accurate, "correct," or it can be caused or modified by systematic errors, imprecision, or both.

A *systematic error* or bias distorts a study in such a way that hypothetical replications of the study would produce the same erroneous result, and a false conclusion would be reached. This type of error has nothing to do with the size of a study, either. Increasing the size of the study would not reduce or eliminate the error. Other measures must be taken to achieve this goal.

A systematic error can be either *positive* or *negative*. In the case of the former, difference is produced between the study groups where there in fact is none or, alternatively, a true difference is exaggerated. When negative, the error masks a true difference partly or completely.

If the study is devoid of systematic error, it is said to be *valid*. Hence "validity" can be defined as the lack of systematic error.

A systematic error distorts the results of a study in such a way that the same average distortion would occur, should the study be repeated.

If there are *random errors* in a study, *imprecision* results. This problem arises if the precision of the measurements is poor; it makes no difference whether the imprecise measurements were of outcome or exposure. This type of imprecision creates scatter due to random variation around the true value. If truly random, errors in outcome measurements (say, blood pressure) level out on an average in large materials, and do not create a false impression of effect when there is none. However, they increase the *variation* of the measurement and thereby produce "background noise." Hence random errors tend to mask a true difference between the populations studied, and give rise to falsely negative, not falsely positive, results. This property is in contrast to that of systematic errors, which may act in either direction.

Random errors due to imprecision level out in a sufficiently large study. They decrease the sensitivity of the study.

Random variation of the point estimate of the summary result of a whole study (e.g., the RR) also causes a kind of imprecision when regarding a set of studies. Then the results, e.g., the $\widehat{RR}$'s, of single studies, given the same magnitude of effect in each study, then vary in the same manner as the results of individual measurements in one particular study. The smaller the study, the larger the random variation. By increasing the study size, investigators can narrow the range within which the study result is likely to vary by chance. Statistical significance tests give some guidance for assessing the likelihood that the result obtained is not within the random distribution that would occur under the null hypothesis (i.e., that no real effect exists), given the study size and the magnitude of the effect. However, as discussed further in Chapter 9, the p-value should be interpreted as a partial summary of the evidence for or against the denial of the study hypothesis, not merely as the probability of the data being due to chance (Reference 26, p. 113). Likewise, the confidence interval of the $\widehat{RR}$ gives a measure of the range of $\widehat{RR}$ values that are consistent with the data. It should be stressed that neither the p-value nor the confidence interval for the rate ratio gives any information at all about the effects of systematic errors.

Generalizability means the potential for extrapolation of the results of a single study, either to a larger "superpopulation," or to the abstract level of scientific theories. Statistical representativeness, which means that the study population is a representative sample of a larger population, is important for a particularistic sample-to-population generalization, whereas scientific representativeness is the foundation for generalization to the abstract-general level. Of course, a study must have high internal validity before either type of generalization is meaningful.

INTERNAL VALIDITY

Systematic errors have traditionally been divided into the three categories: selection bias, information bias, and comparison bias.[5] A more modern approach is to take the clinical trial as the paradigm and to define validity in terms of comparability of effects, of populations, and of information.[26] This being a basic textbook, the traditional view is presented.

Validity of Selection

Selection bias arises whenever the property under study, operationally the exposure in a case-referent design, and the presence or absence of disease in a cohort or exposure-based cross-sectional design, systematically influences whether or not the subjects are chosen into the study.

Example 1. Suppose that the study concerns the prevalence of coronary heart disease (CHD) among viscose rayon workers exposed to carbon disulfide. The occupational health physician could see the investigation as an opportunity for having a free medical check of potentially affected workers. He therefore especially selects workers who have earlier reported symptoms suggestive of CHD for the examination. Suppose also that there is no such tendency in the selection of the reference group. The result is a positive selection bias, leading to overestimation of the effects of carbon disulfide. This error can be easily avoided by not allowing occupational health services to influence the selection of the subjects.

Selection bias is a serious problem in cross-sectional studies. The exposure itself, be it physical load, heat, dustiness, stress, or whatever strain, usually leads to health-selective turnover in the sense that those most affected tend to quit the job. Correspondingly, those remaining are probably more resistant to the effects of the exposure and do not experience too much discomfort from it. Whenever the study is restricted to these "survivors," the result becomes biased, and the true health effects of the exposure in question become underestimated. In other words, the very factors being studied cause the most affected persons to be excluded from the study. There are some empirical results showing that this type of selection may be strong indeed (Figure 1).

Example 2. Suppose we are interested in whether heavy forestry work causes lumbar disorders. If the study design is cross-sectional, the study groups will be selected according to their present job. Suppose that lumberjacks are being compared to a group without similar strain, for example, foresters and foremen. A negative selection bias is inherent in such a design. First, those already suffering from lumbar disease avoid lumbering, because they know well that it is a heavy job. Second, back problems manifested during lumbering force those with symptoms to quit the job. The effects of lumbering work on back pain may, with this study design, become completely or partly masked by such negative selection bias.

Although this example is exaggerated, it is typical, because most knowledge of the interaction between back diseases and work derives from cross-sectional studies (e.g., Reference 9). In spite of this negative selection bias, most of the studies published indicate that heavy physical work causes or exacerbates

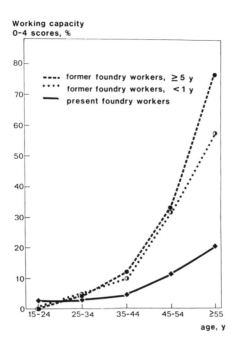

Figure 1. Example of health-based selection. Former and present foundry workers were requested to score their work capacity so that score 10 corresponded to their own best work capacity ever and score 0 to complete inability to work. The figure shows the share of those who considered their present work capacity to be poor (scores 0 to 4). There were big differences between the active and former foundry workers, and the differences became accentuated with advancing age.[17]

back diseases. Hence the true effect of heavy work is probably even greater than that suggested by available results from cross-sectional studies.

Selection bias is a problem in cross-sectional studies.

In case-referent studies, selection bias arises whenever prior knowledge of the exposure in question influences the investigators' selection of cases for the study. In other words, selection validity requires the investigators to be unaware of the exposure histories of the cases and referents when they select the study material. However, there are also other mechanisms for selection bias, especially when the study is based on hospital materials.

Example 3. Suppose we are interested in the hepatotoxicity of organic solvents used as thinners in spray painting. Let us further suppose that the study is carried out at a clinic for occupational medicine. Let the criteria for liver toxicity be repeatedly elevated values of transaminases and a pathological liver biopsy. The cases are then defined according to these preset criteria. The reference group may be a sample of all other patients attending the clinic, matched for age and gender. The exposure history is then collected by a structured interview of the cases and the referents, completed with data obtained from the employer. Exposure to solvents is likely to be more common among the patients having "liver disease." Let us suppose that the $\widehat{OR}$ is 4 (see Table 7, Chapter 2), and that this $\widehat{OR}$ is statistically significant. Superficially this result would indicate that the solvents used in spray painting cause liver damage. However, the truth may be quite different. For a long time many solvents have been suspected of liver toxicity (certain solvents probably rightly so at high doses), and therefore occupational health physicians are probably selective when remitting patients to a clinic of occupational medicine. Those workers who both have elevated transaminases and are exposed to solvents will be remitted more easily than others. For this reason the OR in this example is in error (positive bias), and no conclusions can be drawn from it.

As a rule such a selection bias arises whenever the remitting physician suspects a cause–effect relationship and selectively remits the patients to a specialized center. Therefore the patients seen at any clinic for occupational diseases are strongly selected. Hence the reasons for such selection are:

- There is a specialized center for occupational diseases
- The connection between a certain exposure and certain symptoms and signs is already known or suspected

Several recent well-conducted studies have shown that solvents used as thinners in painting do not cause liver damage under current exposure conditions. Data in the older literature may be different, either because of invalid study design or because of prevailing extremely high exposure levels at the time. Erroneous extrapolation from the effects of high exposure to toxic chlorinated hydrocarbons to lower concentrations of other solvents then creates the false impression that all solvents are hepatotoxic, even at lower levels. The idea that all solvents are hepatotoxic still persists, and the situation could, even in real life, be similar to the one described in the preceding fictitious example.

Selection bias is always a potential source of error in case-referent studies that draw the cases from hospital materials. This source of error is usually called Berkson's fallacy after the epidemiologist who first described it. There are several explanations for certain patients being remitted to or seeking care at certain hospitals. Factors influencing this selection are, among others, the specialization of the hospital (medical field, excellency), geographic factors (different catchment areas for different diseases), and social factors (private vs. general hospitals). These mechanisms vary greatly from one country to another. Therefore, the interpretation of a case-referent study that has drawn its subjects from hospitals, and has been carried out in a foreign country, can be tricky indeed if the authors fail to discuss the local selection mechanisms. In countries with free or very inexpensive medical care, such as the Nordic countries, selection on social grounds is unlikely, but the specialization of different hospitals can still invoke problems. For example, the treatment of some rare disease can be allocated to a few hospitals whose patients otherwise come from a more restricted area. In the United States there are several hospitals having totally different mechanisms of selection, such as expensive private hospitals, Jewish hospitals, veterans' administration hospitals, general hospitals, and so forth. Readers not familiar with the mechanisms determining the selection of patients to each one of them cannot judge the likelihood of selection bias without proper help from the authors.

Selection bias arises in case-referent studies whenever the exposure suspected of causing the outcome influences the selection of cases.

Selection bias is less of a problem in cohort studies. However, occupational health is unfortunately an exception because self-selection rules the choice of occupations or jobs. Health-related causes may influence such decisions to a great extent. Different diseases give rise to different types of health selection, as do different occupations and jobs. Diseases with a long silent latency period are less decisive for job selection than diseases which are affected by occupational strain. For example, persons having chronic bronchitis tend to avoid dusty jobs, and persons with back problems cannot seek physically demanding jobs. Preemployment examinations may accentuate this kind of selection. This so-called healthy worker effect is discussed in more detail later in this chapter.

Later deteriorations of the health state may lead to selection during the course of employment. This type of selection is easier to evaluate because those workers who quit for health reasons can be traced; sometimes they even accept a medical examination. In a qualitative study the effects of negative selection can be avoided in this way. By contrast, if the study is quantitative, this kind of selection leads to underestimation of exposure-related health effects because many of those who should have been classified as "diseased" may have received exposure for short periods only before quitting the job permanently. The most affected individuals may, therefore, have had the shortest exposure, and the least affected the longest exposure.

Selection bias must be minimized at the planning stage of a study because it is difficult if not impossible to control formally at analysis. If selection bias cannot be avoided completely, its direction and strength can be assessed, and its relative effect on the results must be considered informally when the conclusions are drawn. A small selection bias does not invalidate a study completely, provided its effects have been assessed and evaluated. Avoiding selection bias requires thorough awareness of the factors influencing selection into an occupation, the reasons for turnover of the work force, and the mechanisms determining the hospitalization of patients. Thorough knowledge of the study's subject matter is also essential.

Care must be taken to avoid selection bias when a study is planned. Selection bias cannot be formally controlled in the analyses of the results.

Validity of Information

Information bias arises whenever there is *asymmetry* in the quality of information on the study and reference groups. In a case-referent study, the exposure histories of the cases and the referents must be equally accurate (or inaccurate) and equally detailed. Similarly, in cross-sectional and cohort studies, the morbidity of both the exposed and the unexposed groups must be measured with the same accuracy.

Inaccuracy, as such, does not necessarily cause bias, provided it is symmetrical. It is asymmetrical inaccuracy that causes bias, but the *sensitivity* of the study, meaning its power to reveal a true connection between exposure and disease, weakens if the information is symmetrically inaccurate or crude. Low sensitivity may lead to complete or partial masking of the true risk.

Information bias can occur in all study types. It is generally said that the problem is worst in case-referent studies because they largely rely on information gathered by anamnestic data reported in questionnaires and interviews, not on measurements.

Asymmetrical inaccuracy of information causes positive or negative information bias. Symmetrical inaccuracy masks true differences.

The information bias that may occur in a case-referent study has many components, of which three will be presented in this context. The first is connected with the process of recall and it is therefore called *recall bias*. In general people forget even major events (e.g., hospitalizations, operations), not to speak of minor issues. Forgetting as such does not cause bias, but an information bias arises as soon as the cases remember their exposures better than the referents. The illness may have caused them to ponder its possible causes.

The second component has to do with the technique of interviewing. The interviewer may interview cases and referents in different ways, which can result in asymmetrical recall. As an exaggerated example, he or she may ask the case: "You have been exposed to solvents, haven't you?" and the referent: "You haven't had exposure to solvents in your work, have you?" This type of asymmetry is often called *observer bias*.

The third type of information bias has to do with *exaggeration and wrong information* given on purpose. Occupational health problems may be inflamed (e.g., conflicts of interest, compensation claims), and in such situations some cases may succumb to giving false information. Sometimes the issue under study can be hidden among other questions, but sometimes general knowledge is so widespread that this control method fails. The whole research project may then have to be deserted.

> *Example 4.* Suppose that we are interested in whether occupational factors can cause congenital malformations. The cases are mothers of children with malformations, and the referents are mothers of healthy babies. The information is collected in interviews focused on specific exposures during the first trimester of pregnancy, such as intake of medicines, infections, occupational exposures, radiological examinations, use of coffee, tobacco, and alcohol, and the like. The case mothers, who have been brooding over the reasons for their tragedy, are likely to remember their exposures during pregnancy better than the reference mothers, who have had no reason to reflect on such matters. At least minor exposures are likely to be forgotten by the referents. The interviewer may even, knowingly or unknowingly, penetrate the histories of case mothers more deeply. The result may be overreporting, and thus exaggerated OR values for many exposures, especially those which are already known to be teratogenic (e.g., radiological examinations, some medicines). If no prior hypothesis exists, the interpretation of such results is impossible. However, if there is a well-founded, specific prior hypothesis and if only the suspected exposure gives an elevated OR, the result can be interpreted as supporting the view that this exposure is indeed teratogenic.

Although this example illustrates how information bias can arise in a case-referent study, as a rule, there are few empirical data supporting it. People recall some matters better than others. Minor events are probably easier forgotten than major ones, and such events can probably be influenced by asymmetrical recall. Accordingly, cases may be more prone to report use of medicines, minor infections, and other small items than referents. In general, people remember certain major matters well, such as the jobs they have held, or regular matters, such as smoking and the use of alcohol. Therefore the history is assumedly more symmetrical when the subjects are interrogated about such matters. (Even though reported alcohol consumption is known to understate the true consumption severely, there is no a priori reason to assume systematic differences between cases and referents.)

Example 5. Pershagen and Axelson[31] showed that relatives of patients who had died from lung cancer gave an accurate occupational history for them (true positive answers 98%, true negative answers 99% when former employment in a large smelter was the issue). When specific exposure to arsenic was in question, the true positive answers dropped to 40%, but the true negative answers remained as high as 90%. The smoking habits reported by the relatives tallied well with the information noted in the records of the occupational health service.

One study should not be generalized too much, but these results, in fact, do not support the commonly held belief that positive information bias is always a serious problem in case-referent studies.

The occupational setting has an advantage over others because the cases and the referents are not the only potential sources of information. Additional or confirmatory information on the occupational history or even on specific exposures can sometimes be obtained from the employer. This possibility has been utilized in some of the studies carried out by the Finnish Institute of Occupational Health.[10,11,13,18] In these studies experienced occupational hygienists first blindly evaluated the occupational history obtained in an interview and then coded the exposures according to preset criteria (e.g., a specially constructed JEM). Whenever the exposure history indicated the possibility of chemical exposure, they completed and verified the occupational history by contacting the employer, still without knowing whether the person in question was case or a referent. The identification codes were not broken until all the exposure histories were completed. Because most people have an occupational history without any chemical exposure, employer contacts are usually needed for less than 20% of all subjects. Verifying the exposure data with employer interviews improves the quality of information, for example, by providing more details about the specific type of chemical exposure. However, sometimes not even the employer can recall past conditions or exposures, and particularly small companies come and go. If the company is no longer in business, checking the exposure history, of course, is not possible. Such situations especially hamper studies spanning a long time period.

Using the JEM method also improves the validity of the exposure histories. However, such objective methods cannot be used for gathering information on potential confounders, such as smoking and alcohol use.

Potential recall bias can be reduced by means of checking the occupational history with the employer.

Retrospective cohort studies are also vulnerable to information bias because "exposed" groups are usually surveyed more intensively than unexposed ones, for example, by organizing more periodic health examinations for the former categories. Thus company health records may contain more detailed information on workers exposed to potentially harmful agents as compared with unexposed workers. Close surveillance, if well conducted, results in the earlier diagnosis of diseases. In mortality studies, this situation probably causes little error, but whenever other morbidity indicators, for example, sickness retirement, are being studied, the information bias is noteworthy.

> *Example 6.* Suppose that a retrospective cohort study is undertaken to evaluate cancer morbidity in a large company, well known for its traditions in occupational health care. Suppose also that the only reference data available are those of the national cancer register. As far as mortality is concerned, the bias caused by better-than-normal health care, resulting in early detection and perhaps better prognosis for some types of cancer, would cause a negative bias. However, if cancer incidence is being studied as a complement to mortality, the same circumstances could result in earlier detection especially of slow and less malignant forms of cancer, and the bias would be positive.

It must be emphasized that whenever the general population is used as the reference material in a mortality study, causes of death must not be corrected in the exposed cohort even if misdiagnoses are found. In this manner the requirement of symmetry of the information is secured. There is no way to check the national death statistics for diagnostic accuracy, and no way to correct for misdiagnoses in such a reference material. Correcting the causes of death in the exposed group, or excluding misdiagnosed cases, would therefore necessarily be asymmetrical, and hence introduce bias. The usual (wrong) procedure has been to scrutinize the cases of the disease of interest thoroughly, without other diagnoses being considered; this type of revision can have one direction only, namely, negative, which means a seeming lowering of the "true" RR. Using the general population as the reference category inevitably leads to some inaccuracy of information that must be accepted if the advantages offered by this practice are great enough to outweigh the disadvantages (in addition to all the other validity problems inherent in this type of study). But if the reference population is an ad hoc cohort, then all the diagnoses of both groups should be checked, but symmetrically, which requires the pathologist to be unaware of the exposure status of the subject.

However, in case-referent studies the case diagnosis must always be verified as accurately as possible in order to minimize misclassifications. This process does not create asymmetrical information, provided the diagnoses are checked and the "caseness" is defined before the gathering of information starts. By contrast, the reference diagnosis need not be checked as accurately if the hospital can be presumed to have reasonable diagnostic accuracy. The reason for using diseased persons as referents instead of a sample of the base population is to secure symmetrical quality of information, not to study the reference disease. If this fact is borne in mind, it is irrelevant whether or not all the diagnoses are correct. The point is that the referents are ill and experience the study as meaningful.

Information bias arises in cross-sectional studies and in prospective cohort studies (focusing on milder forms of morbidity than deaths) if the morbidity data of the exposed and unexposed groups are gathered in different ways. The reference group must be examined as frequently and as carefully as the exposed group. Because the investigator can influence the gathering of information in both study designs, it should be possible to control information bias provided enough care is taken.

Control of Information Bias

The following list illustrates some of the methods for controlling or avoiding information bias:

1. Measurements should be carefully and regularly calibrated. Sensitive equipment may fail; reagents may become contaminated or old or may precipitate; and so forth.
2. Measurements should be standardized. One should use preset criteria, for example, for reading radiographs, coding electrocardiograms, and classifying exposure data. Experimental conditions must be kept standardized, for example, the temperature of the laboratory during measurements of the conduction velocities of peripheral nerves or during tests of physical work capacity. When classifying results into normal and abnormal, one must always use the same preset criteria (e.g., depression of the S–T interval $\geq$ 1 mm).
3. When serial analyses are run, the proportion of samples from the exposed and unexposed groups must be the same. Minor variations in the accuracy of measurements, for example, from day to day, will then become symmetrically distributed between the groups.
4. Whenever possible, those who perform the measurements and those who interpret them should be blinded. Blinding is possible for laboratory tests, the reading of electrocardiographic films, or roentgenologic examinations. However, as soon as the study embodies oral communication with the subjects (e.g., psychological tests, interviews in case-referent studies), blinding is not feasible.
5. Whenever more than one observer takes part in the study, everyone must be trained to achieve the same accuracy and precision of measurement. In addition, the investigator should assess how well this training has succeeded by measuring the *interobserver error*. The magnitude of the interobserver error can be assessed if different observers perform measurements on the same sample of the subjects and the results are compared. It is rare to succeed in eliminating this error completely. Therefore, the different observers should perform the same proportion of measurements for the different groups under study (i.e., the exposed and the referents, different categories of the exposed). Whenever repeated measurement involves learning on the part of the subjects, first and second measurements should be equally distributed between the observers. The interobserver error should always be given in the study report (but it is unfortunately usually either not measured at all or its reporting has been omitted).

6. Measurements made by the same observer also vary during the course of the study. The more diffuse the parameter to be measured (e.g., early lung fibrosis), the more important the *intraobserver error* because the observer becomes more experienced with time and subconsciously starts applying new or modified criteria. The intraobserver error can also be measured. Its distorting effect can be prevented if the daily proportion of exposed and unexposed subjects for whom measurements are made is kept constant throughout the study. However, in practice, this rule, as simple as it seems, may prove difficult. For example, in a field examination in which the exposed and unexposed subjects are employed by different companies, it is often not practically possible to switch too frequently between the workplaces.

7. Whenever an interview study is concerned, the interviewers must be well trained. All people are not, and will never become, good interviewers. Choosing good interviewers is therefore important. If possible, the study hypothesis should be kept obscured from both the interviewers and the subjects. The interviewers should use a neutral interviewing technique. Cases and referents must be interviewed in exactly the same way. The time used for the interview is a crude measure of how thorough it has been. It should be noted for each subject so that the time spent on the different categories of subjects can be compared. Open questions may sometimes provide the best information. Therefore it may be useful to begin the interview by requesting the subjects to report the matter of interest in their own words (such as: "Describe a typical workday"). However, this type of question is not feasible when the researcher is interested in long time periods. The interviewer's skill also improves during the course of a study. For this reason, cases and referents should be interviewed in the same proportion during all stages of the study. The use of questionnaires eliminates some of these potential errors. However, in general, the quality of the information gained from questionnaires is poorer than from interviews. Hence the gain in terms of more symmetrical information may be insignificant compared with the loss of quality. If the target group is large, cost factors leave no option. The cheaper questionnaire technique is then the only possibility.

8. As already mentioned, one way of securing symmetrical information is to use patients with another disease as referents. However, overcoming information bias by this method may lead to comparison bias or selection bias. The optimal solution is sometimes difficult to find.

9. Even crude information is better than no information at all. Therefore at least the vital status of all members of a cohort should be ascertained; missing information may be asymmetrical. Migration between countries can make this goal difficult to attain, especially in countries employing many "guest" workers with high mobility. When they move back to their native country, often lacking registers, they are easily lost from follow-up. However, sometimes information on the vital status of foreign citizens can be obtained from their native country without problems. Within the Nordic countries such information can be obtained, but many countries in northern Africa, the Middle East, and Latin America cannot provide such data. If the intended cohort contains many guest workers, the study may be doomed to fail from its very beginning, and it would be better not to initiate it at all.

Validity of Comparison

A valid comparison requires that all the groups to be compared are similar in all relevant aspects, except for the properties characterizing the occurrence relation under study. In cohort studies, it is the exposure by which the groups are defined and in case-referent designs the disease whose presence or absence distinguishes the groups. One can say that the reference group should reflect what *would have happened to the exposed,* had there been no exposure.

In experiments, comparability between the study populations as far as their own characteristics are concerned (such as heredity, concomitant diseases, psychological properties) is best achieved if the subjects (or animals) are randomized into exposed and unexposed groups. Comparability of the study populations means that these populations must be similar with respect to their own characteristics; the index and reference subjects must be "alike," for example, with regard to properties leading to their entry and exit from specific employments, social structure, and all other relevant aspects as well. In epidemiologic studies, randomization is almost never possible. Therefore comparability between the study populations must be achieved through the *choice* of a reference group that secures acceptable comparability.[26]

In clinical trials, comparability of the effects to be studied (e.g., the efficacy of a treatmnent) is achieved through the use of a placebo or another treatment (usually the "conventional" treatment) for the control group. In epidemiologic research, the exposed group should be compared to a reference group without the exposure of interest, but with an exposure pattern otherwise similar to that of the study group. Consequently "nonexposure" does not simply mean the absence of exposure, but comparability with respect to other exposures as well.[26] It is therefore important to conceptualize and define the exact issue that the study should address. Is it a specific exposure, a combination of exposures, or something else? For example, if the effects of carbon disulfide on coronary morbidity is the issue, the reference category should be similar in all other respects (such as other chemical exposures, occurrence of shift work, physical strain, and nonoccupational exposures). If, on the other hand, the issue is the combined effects of work in a viscose factory, the reference group should be free from all the characteristics of that work, but similar with respect to nonoccupational exposures, such as tobacco smoking.

This requirement means that most "unexposed" people are not qualified to be valid referents. Only very few of them comply with the requirement of comparability of effects.[26]

The reference group should describe what would have happened to the exposed group, had there been no exposure.

Ideal reference groups are hard to find; therefore, one usually has to compromise. In doing so, one should focus on those population and exposure characteristics that could most likely distort the results of the study. In the realm of occupational health, of the population characteristics at least age should be equally distributed across the groups. One would also be reluctant to neglect the gender distribution. If the number of either the men or the women is too few, the study is better restricted to best represented gender only. Social class is a strong determinant of mortality, and, unless this very effect is being studied, the groups should have a similar social structure. In general, the properties of the populations to be considered depend on the nature of the problem.

The control of external determinants of the disease under study, meaning other exposures, also depends on the nature of the problem. For example, in a study on the relationship between exposure to a foundry environment and lung cancer incidence, one would preferably use a reference group with smoking habits similar to the exposed group's, or carry out the comparisons between subgroups with similar smoking habits. On the other hand, if the issue is the relationship between exposure to chlorinated solvents and primary liver cancer, smoking is not known to be a major risk factor of this disease, whereas consumption of alcohol probably is. Therefore, it is not so relevant to control for smoking in this situation, whereas control for alcohol consumption warrants closer attention. However, as scientific knowledge grows, factors presently unknown to be connected with a disease may later prove to be so. Therefore it may be prudent (if the budget permits) to measure, for possible future control, also some properties of the study groups that presently are not considered risk factors of the disease.

Example 7. The aim of the Finnish carbon disulfide study (see Example 16, Chapter 2 and Example 14, Chapter 4) was to investigate whether the morbidity of coronary heart disease (CHD) was increased by exposure to this substance. The exposed group was formed of workers who had been employed by a viscose rayon plant for at least 5 years, and the reference group of workers with similar employment in a nearby paper mill. It was assumed that the work environment in both plants (disregarding the exposure to carbon disulfide) had the same effect, if any, on the risk of developing CHD. Both plants were process in-

Table 1. Achievement of Comparability between the Exposed and the Reference Group

Characteristic	Method	Similarity
Age	Pair-matching	Same
Gender	Restriction	Males only
Minimum employment	Restriction	Same
Birth district	Pair-matching	Same
Type of work	Pair-matching	Same
Social structure	Result of matching	Same
District of habitation	Questionnaire	Same
Cigarette consumption	Questionnaire	No major differences
Leisure-time physical activity	Questionnaire	No major differences
Physical work capacity	Ergometry	No major differences
Relative body weight	Measurement	Same
Drug therapy	Questionnaire	No major differences
Diet	Judgment	No major differences

Source: Hernberg et al.[12]

dustries, noise levels were high in both, high temperatures occurred in several jobs in both, shift work was typical of both, and both had the same distribution of tasks with regard to blue- or white-collar jobs. Some other chemical exposures occurred, different in each of the plants, but none was known or suspected of being cardiotoxic. Hence, the work environments were comparable. Equally important was to ensure comparability of the populations with respect to the major coronary risk factors (known in 1967). These were age, gender, birth district, leisure-time physical activity, area of habitation, and social class. Because only some 20 women had been exposed, it was decided to restrict the study to men only. Table 1 summarizes how the most important coronary risk factors were measured and controlled. The groups were not matched for blood lipids, blood pressure, or fasting blood glucose level (which were all measured, though) because according to the literature, it was possible that the cardiotoxic effect of carbon disulfide might have been transmitted through any one of these mechanisms, or all of them. One should never match on intermediate steps in the causal chain from cause to effect because such a procedure would mask the true effect exerted by the exposure.[26]

Now, with more than 20 years of additional experience with occupational cohort studies, one would hardly consider individual matching because of the vast effort involved. Practical difficulties could easily arise in finding referents if the reference pool were not very ample. Fortunately, there was a surplus of potential referents in the paper mill, and sufficient technical assistance was available. Although the matching procedure was cumbersome (it took 6 weeks), a referent could be found for every exposed subject. The result of the matching was not only better comparability of the groups, but also improved efficiency of the study, because all subsets of the population became balanced.

Those not familiar with the epidemiology of CHD in Finland may wonder why the region of birth was matched for. CHD was (especially in those days) more frequent in eastern than in western Finland. It was known beforehand that when the plant, originally founded in Karelia, was evacuated to western Finland during World War II, all of its workers also migrated. The result was that 40% of the workers employed by the viscose rayon plant in 1967 had been born in Karelia, whereas only 25% of the paper mill workers were of Karelian origin.

Individual matching was by no means the only option with which to control the asymmetry of the birth district. Matched stratified sampling or other methods could well have been used, such as stratifying for birth district at analysis. (Modeling was not yet commonplace in the early 1970s.) Irrespective of the method chosen, the matter could not be neglected, because the coronary mortality in eastern Finland was known to be about 50% higher than in western Finland in those days. Today modeling in the data analysis would be the method of choice for controlling this confounding effect. Be it as it may, this example illustrates how important it is for epidemiologists to know their subject matter well.

In a *case-referent study*, in which patients with a disease other than the index disease are used as referents, a comparison bias may arise if the disease is not completely independent of the exposure(s) under study. The referents should provide an estimate of the exposure distribution in the study base, and this estimate would be incorrect if the reference disease is either caused or prevented by the exposure under study. Choosing a "neutral" disease as the reference disease is therefore important. The problem is that the effects of many exposures are unknown. When several potential causes for a disease are being studied, a reference disease, which is neither caused nor prevented by any of them, may be difficult to find.

In case-referent studies, the reference group shows the exposure pattern in the whole study base or alternatively, among the noncases.

Example 8. In the Nordic case-referent study on nasal and sinonasal cancer (see Example 14, Chapter 4), patients with colonic cancer were chosen as referents.[13] The assumption was that none of the studied exposures caused or prevented this cancer form. Had only one exposure been the issue, selecting a reference cancer would have been easier. However this study was partly open-ended in the sense that, apart from wood dust, other exposures were also studied. Of the exposures studied, wood dust, nickel, and chromates are not suspected of causing colonic cancer. This statement cannot be made of asbestos, whose relation to nasal cancer would have been interesting to explore. Because it has been suggested that asbestos may cause colonic cancer, this reference category was not suitable for exploring the etiologic role of asbestos. Therefore the Nordic nasal cancer study was uninformative in this respect.

Confounding

Confounding can occur when the researcher has not succeeded in finding a reference group that is comparable with the index group with regard to

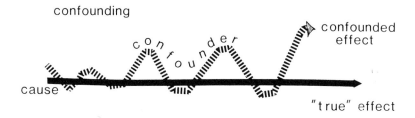

Figure 2. A confounding factor is intermixed with the problem under study. It distorts the true relation between exposure and outcome.

intrinsic or extrinsic relevant characteristics. The word "relevant" means those characteristics that are predictive of risk among people in general, such as age, gender, and certain biochemical characteristics (intrinsic), as well as life-style factors (diet and smoking are examples), other chemical exposures, and shift work (extrinsic). If the study groups are not comparable in such respects, that is, if these or other risk factors are asymmetrically distributed, there will be confounding. Thus a *confounding factor* is an extraneous determinant of the outcome parameter that is asymmetrically distributed between the index group and the reference group. A confounding factor distorts the occurrence relation of interest (Figure 2).

As a rule of thumb one can thus say that a confounding factor is characterized by the following two properties:

1. It is a *causal* risk factor of the disease under study
2. It is correlated to the exposure in the *particular study* (without being a consequence of the exposure)

In other words, if a causal risk factor of the disease (other than the one under study) occurs more (or less) frequently among the exposed than among the referents, the study is confounded. The connection to the disease must always be causal, meaning that a confounder must be a true risk factor of the disease, whereas the relation to the exposure does not need to be causal. It may occur in one study but not in another.

Example 9. Consider a study exploring whether dust exposure causes chronic bronchitis. Smoking (which is always a causal risk factor for bronchitis) is a confounder only if the exposed group contains more (or less) smokers than the reference group. This situation may occur in a particular study, whereas another may have a symmetrical distribution of smokers in both groups. In the former instance smoking *is* a confounder, in the latter it is *not*.

Example 10. Consider another study investigating the effect of smoking on the occurrence of lung cancer. It has been observed that smokers have yellow fingers more often than nonsmokers. Patients with lung cancer also have yellow fingers more frequently than other patients. Is the property of having yellow fingers a confounding factor?

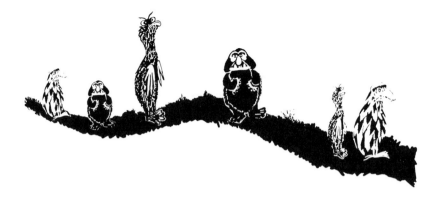

Figure 3. A confounder is not always the same-looking, easily identifiable monster.

As already stated, a confounder must *both* be a causal risk factor of the disease *and* be statistically associated with the exposure. In this case, yellow fingers are indeed related to the exposure, because smoking often results in discoloration of the fingers. Hence one of the requirements is met. The relation to lung cancer is, on the other hand, not causal, because yellow fingers as such do not cause lung cancer. Likewise, getting rid of the yellow color by using a strong detergent, or even amputation for that sake, does not reduce the cancer risk. The connection to lung cancer is clearly noncausal. Hence having yellow fingers cannot be a true confounder, although this property is a nonspecific indicator of smoking. It could be considered a proxy for an exposure parameter of smoking.

A causal risk factor of a disease is typically a confounder if it occurs more or less frequently among the exposed in a particular study.

The previous text and Examples 9 and 10 underline the fact that a confounder is not a sort of monster that always looks the same and is easily identified (Figure 3).

Instead, confounders are intermixed with the problem in question. The same factor can sometimes be and at other times not be a confounder (Figure 4). It is the intermixing that decides whether a risk factor becomes a confounder or not. The identification of a confounder requires thorough consideration and good knowledge of the subject matter. Age, smoking, drinking, and the like are not automatically confounders. In some situations they may confound the study, while in others they do not.

If a confounding factor distorts a study, its strength is unique to that study. It depends on how asymmetrically the confounder is distributed across the

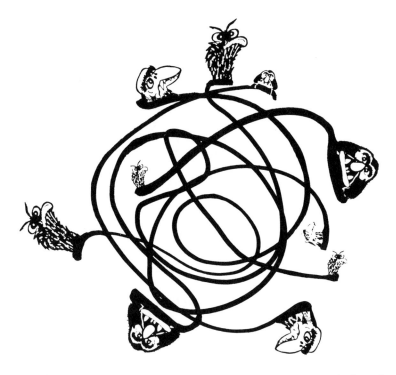

Figure 4. Confounders, although they may be ugly, even when alone, must be intermixed with the problem in order to fulfill the criteria for confounding.

exposed and reference categories. In another study the confounding effect of the same factor may be stronger or weaker; it may even shift from positive to negative. This variation is not random (such as the estimate of the RR in small studies), but depends on the degree of asymmetry in each particular study. Therefore one should not apply statistical testing to help decide whether there is confounding if a difference between the distribution of a confounding factor (say, smoking) among the study groups has been observed. The strength of the confounding effect depends on how large the difference is in the study in question. It has nothing to do with whether or not the result was due to chance. For example, if smoking occurs 15% more frequently among the exposed persons in a study on the work-relatedness of CHD, its confounding effect is exactly what 15% more smoking gives rise to in terms of CHD in that particular study. It is totally irrelevant if the 15% difference is ''significant'' or not. In another study the difference could turn out to be something else, depending on the smoking habits of the particular populations of this study. Moreover, a difference of 15% could be statistically nonsignificant in a small study, whereas even a 5% difference could be ''significant'' in a large study. If only ''significance'' were to decide whether smoking is a confounder, the larger difference would be left without control in the data analysis, while the smaller one would be adjusted for. Such a practice, of course, would be nonsense.

Example 11. The Finnish study on carbon disulfide, referred to earlier, showed an excess of both fatal and nonfatal coronary infarctions in the exposed group. Could smoking have been a confounder?

Smoking is a causal risk factor of CHD; hence, it fulfills one of the requirements for confounding. In order to fulfill the other, it should be associated with the exposure in that particular study or smoking should be more (or less) common among the exposed workers than among the referents. In general, the smoking habits are not known when the study groups are selected, so this information must be gathered in connection with the study, usually by a self-administered questionnaire or an interview. If smoking then turns out to be asymmetrically distributed across the groups, it must be controlled as a confounder in the data analysis. If not, smoking does not fulfill the second requirement for a confounder and does not require control in the analysis, which may seem surprising at first sight. In this example, the questionnaire revealed that the asymmetry of smoking habits was so slight that smoking could not confound the relation between exposure to carbon disulfide and the incidence of coronary attacks to any remarkable degree. Hence smoking was not treated as a confounder in the data analysis.

However, there is another reason to scrutinize different smoking categories separately. Smoking could be an *effect modifier* for the relation between carbon disulfide exposure and CHD, meaning that the effect could be stronger for heavy smokers (or weaker, but this is not biologically plausible in our example). Scrutinizing such possible effect modification could help shed more light on the mechanism whereby carbon disulfide contributes to the causation of CHD. For this reason the $\widehat{RR}$ was separately computed for different smoking categories. There was no difference, that is, the $\widehat{RR}$ was similarly elevated in all smoking categories (as far as conclusions can be drawn from the small numbers in the subcategories).

Confounding can cause both qualitative and quantitative distortions, quite like other biases. Positive confounding either gives rise to a false difference where there should be none or exaggerates a true effect. Negative confounding either masks a true effect completely or decreases it. If the true effect is weak only, confounding can turn a positive effect into a negative one, and vice versa.

Example 12. Suppose that the exposed workers in the previous example for some reason had *underreported* their smoking systematically. Such underreporting would have caused an information bias affecting a *potential confounder*. Consequently, the seeming symmetry of smoking habits would have been false, or the exposed group would, in fact, have smoked more than the reference group. Then smoking would have been an undetected positive confounder, unaccounted for—and unaccountable—in the analysis. When considering such possibilities, one should apply common sense: is there some specific reason why only the exposed subjects would underreport smoking? If no good reason can be found, why should one a priori assume such a distortion? And even if this explanation would be well founded, how much of the excess risk could be

Table 2. Estimated Crude Rate Ratios (RR) in Relation to the Fraction of Smokers in Various Hypothetical Populations[a]

Population Fraction (%)			
Nonsmokers (1×)	Moderate Smokers (10×)	Heavy Smokers (20×)	RR
100	—	—	0.15
80	20	—	0.43
70	30	—	0.57
60	35	5	0.78
50	40	10	1.00[b]
40	45	15	1.22
30	50	20	1.43
20	55	25	1.65
10	60	30	1.86
—	65	35	2.08
—	25	75	2.69
—	—	100	3.08

[a] Two different risk levels are assumed for smokers, i.e., 10 and 20 times that of nonsmokers for "moderate" and "heavy" smokers, respectively (from Axelson[4]).
[b] Reference population (similar to the general population in countries like Sweden). Smoking habits in various industrial populations rarely diverge outside the dotted lines.

explained by confounding? The phenomenon of confounding is not black and white. Confounding should also be viewed in quantitative terms. By this token, totally explaining away an RR with a point estimate of 4.7 by confounding, as in the example, would not be credible.

Confounding can be either positive or negative.

In occupational epidemiology, confounding by nonoccupational external factors is perhaps not such a serious problem as generally believed. Axelson[4] has estimated theoretically the extent to which different degrees of asymmetry in smoking habits can confound the true RR for lung cancer (Table 2). His intention was to give some estimate of how much confounding could distort the point estimate of the "true" RR in a study in which the smoking habits of the exposed cohort were not known to the investigator. In his hypothetical example he used the general male Swedish population as the reference category. His estimation of its smoking habits was based on a survey done some years earlier in Sweden. Other general populations may have different smoking habits than the Swedish one, but this point is not relevant as long as the comparisons are made within one country. The message of this exercise is that the asymmetry must be rather extreme to cause any substantial distortion of the true RR. The explanation is, of course, that smokers are not compared to nonsmokers, but to a population distributing a certain pattern of smoking habits.

Table 3. Estimated Rate Ratios (RR) of Lung Cancer in Relation to the Percentage of Nonsmokers, Ex-smokers, and Smokers in Various Occupational Groups[a]

Occupational Group	Percentage of Group			Estimated RR
	Nonsmokers (RR = 1)	Ex-smokers (RR = 10)	Smokers (RR = 20)	
Least proportion of smokers				
Civil servants	41	37	22	0.67
Business executives	30	40	30	0.81
Scientific and engineering personnel	27	37	36	0.88
. . . .				
Total study population	24	28	48	1.00
. . . .				
Greatest proportion of smokers				
Miners and workers in the basic metal industry	20	17	63	1.15
Packers, loaders and depot workers	13	22	65	1.21
Operators of mobile machines	7	25	68	1.28
Construction workers	10	16	74	1.31

[a] On the assumption of RR = 1 for the whole sample, a 20-fold risk for smokers, and a 10-fold risk for ex-smokers. The assumed risks for smokers and ex-smokers are extreme; hence, the results exaggerate the effect of smoking.

In Table 2 it is assumed that 50% of the general population comprises ex-smokers or nonsmokers, 40% smokes moderately, and 10% smokes heavily. The other assumption is that the risk of developing lung cancer is 20-fold for heavy smokers and 10-fold for moderate smokers, as compared with the risk of nonsmokers (including ex-smokers). Even if an exposed group would contain 20% heavy smokers and only 30% nonsmokers, the confounding effect of smoking on the point estimate of the RR would be no more than 1.43-fold.

In conclusion, Axelson's exercise shows that the possible confounding effect of smoking is weaker than generally believed in studies of work-related lung cancer with the general population as the reference category. However, his calculations apply to crude, unstandardized rates only.

These assumptions have been applied empirically by Asp,[3] who gathered information on the smoking habits of a sample of 1990 Finnish men. She used Axelson's assumptions to estimate how much the observed differences in smoking habits would have confounded a hypothetical $\widehat{RR}$ for lung cancer on the assumption that this disease otherwise would have been equally distributed in the different occupational categories (Table 3). As compared with the average smoking frequency in the sample (which was probably a good estimate of the Finnish male population), the confounded point estimate of the RR varied only between 0.7 and 1.3, although Asp used rather extreme assumptions. Both Axelson's theoretical calculations and Asp's empirical data clearly show that smoking can be a practically significant confounder only when the observed $\widehat{RR}$ for lung cancer is between 0.5 and 2.0. Such values are by no means rare in studies on work-related lung cancer, so the problem should not be neglected. However, confounding by smoking cannot explain higher observed $\widehat{RR}$ values, at least not completely. Consequently, a study showing an $\widehat{RR}$ of, say, 3.5, cannot be invalidated only because data on smoking were not available.

If the confounding effect of smoking in studies on work-related lung cancer has sometimes been exaggerated, the possible effects of other previous or concomitant occupational exposures have received too little attention.

Complex and mixed exposure patterns usually render the epidemiologic identification of a specific causative agent impossible. In less complicated situations combined exposures require very thorough exposure histories and adequate data analysis. Sometimes even these measures are insufficient, and the identification of the carcinogen (or whatever agent causing some chronic disease) must rely on other types of data than epidemiologic data.

> *Example 13.* An excess of leukemia was observed among workers in an American styrene-butadiene rubber plant.[24] Exposure to both styrene and butadiene occurred in almost all the jobs. It was not possible to determine which agent was causative with respect to the observed excess of leukemia.

Control of Confounding

A confounding factor can be controlled either in the planning of a study or at the data analysis stage, as stated before. *Randomization* is the most effective method of controlling confounding. It is the method of choice in clinical trials and other experimental work. Randomization means that the study subjects are randomly allocated into exposed and unexposed groups. However, if the groups are small, it is likely that some degree of confounding remains or even arises due to chance. In other words, the randomization can result in an unbalanced distribution of risk factors between the groups. Unfortunately, randomization is rarely if ever possible in epidemiologic studies. Therefore confounding must be controlled by other methods.

The methods for controlling confounding in epidemiologic studies are restriction, matching, standardization, stratification, and modeling.

Restriction means that the study is focused on one category only, for example, the age group 40 to 69 years, only men, only nonsmokers, only those exposed for more than 20 years, only those without mixed exposure, and so forth. The study material can further be restricted so that the distribution of potential confounders becomes as symmetrical as possible in both groups (cf. frequency matching), if "surplus" individuals are removed. The groups can, for example, be so selected that they contain 30% white collar workers, 50% nonsmokers, a balanced age distribution, and so on. Such restriction improves the comparability of the groups. Often restriction is used to increase the *efficiency* of the study rather than to control confounding, for example, the exclusion of categories with low morbidity or with multiple exposures. Improving efficiency saves work and funds. The issue is to find a category for which the effect is largest in relation to the "background noise." In other words, one should not focus only on categories having high incidence, such as elderly people in a study on cerebrovascular incidents; one should also consider for what category of people the RR is likely to be the highest. This consideration could, for example, lead to rather young men being preferable to older ones in a study on work-related lung cancer.

Restriction alone is a weak method for controlling confounding, especially if the categories are broad. It is therefore usually combined with other methods.

In *matching,* cases and referents are selected so that they are comparable with respect to some potential confounder, such as age, gender, vital status, smoking habits, and time of diagnosis. If matching is performed subject-by-subject, it is called individual matching. If it is performed for groups of subjects, one speaks of frequency matching. It is, for example, not necessary to choose a referent of similar age for each case. Instead, the referents can be so selected that the age distribution of the cases and referents is similar in 10-year intervals (cf. restriction). There are also several other variations of matching.

Matching can be made with respect to one or several factors. The more factors to be matched, the more difficult to find referents, especially if the reference material is restricted. Matching always demands a lot of work, and for this reason should not be used indiscriminantly. Matching is typical of the case-referent design. Although usually effective in terms of unit information per subject, it is, in general, too costly for cohort studies, and it is therefore rarely used. (The carbon disulfide cohort study described in several of the examples was an exception.)

The purpose of matching is to control confounding by the factors that are being matched. Superficially regarded, matching seems conceptually simple. However, this concept is deceptive. In cohort studies, which resemble experiments, the matter is straightforward, and matching can really control confounding. This is not so in case-referent studies, the very domain in which matching is usually employed. Instead of controlling confounding, matching can *introduce* it, if the matching factor is related to the actual exposure.[26,32] To comply with the criteria for a confounder, such a factor should be associated with the exposure. Therefore matching for a true confounder would always introduce confounding, although the type of confounding may be different. The confounding in the study base may have been positive, while matching introduces negative confounding (confounding brought about by matching always being negative). If, on the other hand, the matching factor is not correlated with exposure, matching does not introduce confounding. However, if this indeed is the situation, the factor is, in fact, no confounder (a confounder should be related both to the exposure and to the outcome), and then matching is irrelevant. The problem is that one does not always know beforehand whether or not a risk factor of the disease is associated with the exposure in that particular study, that is, whether or not it is a true confounder.

Matching can introduce negative confounding in case-referent studies.

Matching can be combined with other procedures to control confounding. One can, for example, match on one or two factors only — such as time of case occurrence — and control the rest in the statistical analysis. The current tendency is to be rather restrictive with matching and instead rely on other methods to control confounding, such as modeling. Because matching, instead of controlling confounding, may introduce negative confounding, it is necessary to adjust for it in the analyses. Under no circumstances should one match for a factor that is (or may be) an intermediate in the causal chain between exposure and outcome. Such matching would always tend to mask a true effect, and thereby create a negative bias.[25]

However, although the main motive for matching is to increase the validity of the study — especially the avoidance of positive confounding — matching can also be used to increase its efficiency. Matching ensures a sufficient number of observations in each category of the confounder, and thus it improves the cost-efficiency of the study.

Standardization is usually employed when an exposed cohort is compared to the general population, or when two or more general populations are being mutually compared. The most common stardardized measure is the SMR (see Chapter 2).

Stratification can either be used alone or combined with restriction or matching. Stratification means that the study groups are divided into subgroups or strata on the basis of the confounders to be controlled, for example, age, gender, smoking category, and body weight. Comparisons are then made within the strata. Analysis by stratification controls the effects of the asymmetrical distribution of a risk factor by focusing the comparison on subgroups that are similar with respect to the potential confounder. The entire material can then be recombined, and a summary $\widehat{RR}$ can be computed from the stratum-specific $\widehat{RR}$ values, for example, by the method first developed by Mantel and Haenszel.[20] However, stratification is not effective if the asymmetry is extreme (extreme asymmetry should be avoided at the planning stage through restriction of the study material) because the tails of the distributions are uninformative in that they have no counterpart in the other group.

Table 4. Age Stratification of Two Hypothetical Populations[a]

	Exposed Group		Reference Group	
Age (years)	N	Cases	N	Cases
—19	1	—	38	3
20—29	6	1	97	9
30—39	82	12	124	14
40—49	143	23	158	22
50—59	116	22	59	9
60—69	86	42	8	3
70—	51	39	1	—
Total	485	139	485	60

[a] Because the age distribution is highly asymmetrical, the age groups below 30 and over 60 years are uninformative.

Example 14. Suppose that the age distributions of two populations that are being compared are as asymmetric as those shown in Table 4. The crude $\widehat{RR}$ for the tentative disease is 139/60 = 2.32. However, it is evident that this $\widehat{RR}$ is a strongly biased measure. A stratified analysis will yield a weighted $\widehat{RR}$ of 1.21 (not statistically significant). The bulk of information comes from the age category 30 to 59 years. It remains unsolved whether the high morbidity in the older exposed strata is a consequence of the exposure or if it is "natural."

If stratification is used, the potential confounder must be classified. By this token, a continuous variable (e.g., serum cholesterol value) must be classified either as high, medium or low, or in categories of, say, 1 mmol/L. The more variables to be stratified, the more strata. Thus a stratified analysis requires large study materials. In addition, those with a "high high value" and a "low high value" fall in the same stratum, and therefore confounding by that factor can be only partially controlled. Because problems always arise when stratification is done for many factors, one should, at the planning stage of the investigation, consider seriously if stratification is the best method for controlling confounding. If stratification seems attractive, one should also consider which potential confounders should be controlled by this method and which ones by some other. The extent to which stratification is used in the data analysis is strongly determined by the size of the study material. The more strata, the larger a material required.

Modeling is the method of choice whenever there are several factors to be controlled in the analyses. Greenland[8] defines statistical modeling as "using the data to select an explicit mathematical model for the data-generating process (p. 340)." Model building involves specification of the model form (e.g., logistic), selection of the subject variables (characteristics) to enter the model, and choice of their statistical representation (e.g., indicator) in the model function.

The main advantages of multivariate modeling of epidemiologic data are the possibilities to control more potential confounders than what could be achieved in stratified analysis (in which the strata may run out of numbers if many variables are to be stratified) and to estimate variation in the effect of exposure levels more precisely across levels of other factors (effect modification). For example, is the effect of carbon disulfide exposure on coronary mortality different in different categories of smoking, blood pressure, and serum lipids? The disadvantages of modeling are that strong statistical assumptions, such as equal individual response probabilities within exposure and covariate levels, and independent responses across individuals are required. Therefore efficient use of modeling is more demanding than simple stratified analysis because the correctness of the assumptions must be checked. It will also be more difficult to interpret and understandably present the results from modeling. A reasonable approach is first to reproduce the results of stratified analysis using a few variates to verify the assumptions and only then to enlarge the model to describe and summarize a multivariate dataset. Finally, any available prior information should be used to assess carefully the epidemiologic implications inferred from the chosen model for disease risk.

Modeling is best suited for the control of several factors in a material with many categories.

Healthy Worker Effect

The healthy worker effect (HWE) has been ''scientified'' and treated like an interesting epidemiologic phenomenon in numerous articles, symposia, and, quite recently, in a monograph dedicated to the evaluation of the effects of this distortion on the interpretation of cohort studies.[14] Yet, it is nothing more than a trivial bias, as Miettinen[27] says, ''a manifestation of the benightedness that still shrouds epidemiologic research modeled after its traditional paradigms (p. 72).'' In a cohort study, the reference group should give an estimate of the morbidity in the exposed group, had there been no exposure. However, ''non-exposure should not generally be taken as the absence of exposure (p. 30);''[26] the groups should also be comparable in all other relevant aspects. The vast majority of the general population does not fulfill the latter criterion; only a small subset of it may, in fact, be comparable to the exposed cohort. To further quote Miettinen:[26] ''those not meeting the criteria for either the index or the reference category fall in a third, 'other,' category of the determinant (p. 30).''

It is this third ''other'' category that makes up most of the general population. In the light of these considerations, occupational epidemiologists should seek other solutions than to continue persistently to employ a design so fundamentally biased. As Wang and Miettinen[35] ironically describe the problem: ''If therapeutic research were conducted in an analogous manner, treated

Table 5. Some examples of SMR Values Reflecting the HWE[a]

Occupational Category	SMR
Finnish foundry workers[16]	90
"Typical" foundry occupations	95
American steel workers[19]	82
American rubber workers[23]	87
Finnish granite workers[1]	83
Finnish dock workers[2]	81
American chemical workers[30]	81

[a] General population = 100.

patients would be compared with the 'general population' for any criterion of outcome. Experience would show that the treated group usually has a worse outcome than the reference population, and the difference might be referred to as the 'sick patient effect' (p. 153).''

The only plausible explanation for the continuation of this malpractice (to which most of us have unfortunately succumbed) is that mortality figures for the general population are easily available, inexpensive, and stable. The last-mentioned property increases the statistical power of the comparison. However, the time has now come to consider abandoning the old routine of contrasting occupational cohorts to the general population because there are indeed other workable options. (See the later discussion.) But since rather few signs of improvement can be seen even in the most recent epidemiologic literature, a brief discussion of the anatomy of the HWE cannot be avoided in any textbook on occupational epidemiology.

McMichael, who probably can be credited for the labeling of this term,[21] has recently redefined the HWE in the following way:[22]

The HWE refers to the consistent tendency for the actively employed people to have a more favourable mortality experience than the population at large. Despite the clarity seemingly implicit in its name, the HWE is *not* an intentional measurement of the relatively good health of a working population; *nor* does it quantify the beneficial effects of the occupational environment upon those working within it. Rather it is an unintended bias, of uncertain magnitude, in an unavoidably imperfect comparative measure of the health status of a working population (p. 58).

The HWE results in the SMR for the total mortality of an exposed cohort being well below 100, provided there are no work-related or social factors increasing the mortality. In other words, the *HWE is a negative bias*. The literature is full of examples illustrating this phenomenon (e.g., Table 5).

These and other employed populations have a better-than-expected outcome because of the incomparability of the large "third category" of the general population, which contains unemployed, disabled, and asocial people, all of whom have a higher than "normal" mortality. In addition, the general population and a cohort of blue-collar workers differ as to social structure. That this difference has an impact on mortality was well illustrated by Kitagawa and Hauser's survey,[15] which demonstrated that the SMR for unemployed Americans born in 1950 or later (4.3% of the population) was 204. In addition, the SMR of that 4% of the population which had no occupation was 125. Results from a Finnish population survey corroborate these findings.[33]

Even when the SMR for all causes is below 100, some cause-specific SMR may be well above this figure. A low overall SMR therefore does not exclude the possibility of life-shortening exposures occurring in a work environment. It would indeed be hard to think of any occupational factor increasing all causes of death in an equal manner. Therefore the overall SMR reflects social rather than occupational factors (besides bias, of course). However, there are also studies showing that the SMR for all causes of death in occupational cohorts may well be in excess of 100. Usually the reason is a substantial excess of some major single cause of death, such as lung cancer, but, if the cohort comprises many workers belonging to low social categories, the result may be a generally increased mortality as compared with that of the average general population. For example, the SMR of heavily exposed asbestos workers was nearly 200 in a British study, but the increased mortality was due to malignancies, mostly of the lung and pleura, not to an even increase of all causes of death.[29]

The HWE-induced bias has a complex nature. As already stated, it has nothing to do with any beneficial effect of the work environment on the health of the workers. Health-based selection into a certain employment, or into the entire work force for that sake, is the most important cause of the HWE. Merely being fit to work, becoming employed, and subsequently remaining employed give the worker a better than average life expectancy. In addition to this general rule, there are variations between different jobs, those with higher physical demands also having higher demands for health. The correct comparison category for any employed group should be workers with equal work demands and equal a priori health status, not the large third "other" category of the general population. There is also health-based selection out of jobs, which causes more bias the less successfully those leaving the job are traced and their vital status is ascertained. On an average these workers often have poorer health than those remaining.[7,17]

Although there undoubtedly occurs health-based selection into and out of occupations, the bias referred to as the HWE is better regarded as confounding. Confounding is a characteristic of the study population, either intrinsic or extrinsic, or both, while selection bias is a result of the actions of the investigator.[28] The HWE confounding arises from the biased comparison to a noncomparable reference category, the general population, as discussed earlier. The distinction is not only academic, because, in principle, confounding can be controlled during the analyses, while selection bias cannot. However, for the HWE, the main confounding factor, the initial health status, can seldom be measured in an occupational cohort, and never in the entire general population. The same is true for other potential confounders, such as life-style factors, other occupational exposures, and so forth.

Because systematic errors are involved, it is meaningless (although very common) to test deviating SMR values statistically for significance, irrespective of whether they are high or low. It is true that the point estimate of the SMR, in addition to a possible bias has a range of random variation, and according to conventional thinking significance testing assesses the likelihood for the result to be due to chance. (Not even this statement is entirely correct; see the discussion later in this chapter.) To get an idea of the magnitude of variation in the point estimate of the SMR in hypothetical replications of a study, one should check the confidence interval rather than the "black or white" p-value. Neither the confidence interval nor the p-value give any information on systematical errors such as the HWE, however.

The HWE is not constant, but varies due to the following factors:[21,22,28]

1. The HWE is strongest in young age groups, decreases with advancing age, and disappears after retirement. In the case of employed young people, the comparison is with a young general population, including those with congenital defects, mental retardation, and so forth, all of whom have an increased mortality. Workers retired due to old age, again, are not much different from those in the general population who have survived to that age.

2. The HWE is stronger for men than for women, since the female general population includes many women who are inactive for reasons other than health.

3. High social categories show a stronger HWE than low ones because mortality in general is comparatively low in the high social classes. Thus, whenever employed white-collar workers are being compared to a general population whose majority belongs to lower social categories, there must be a strong HWE on social grounds.

4. The HWE is stronger at the beginning of employment, or soon after entrance into a cohort, because health-based selection operates at its strongest at that point.

5. The HWE is different for different causes of death. In general, diseases with a silent early stage and a later rapid course cause an HWE only during the very first years after cohort identification. Cancer is a typical example. With few exceptions, no good methods exist for screening or for such early diagnosis that would significantly improve the prognosis on a group basis, at least not methods applicable in the occupational health service setting. By contrast, a high risk for heart disease can often (although not always) be diagnosed years in advance, either as early manifestations of coronary insufficiency or as the presence of coronary risk factors (e.g., hypertension, high serum cholesterol, heavy smoking). In addition, early symptoms of the disease, such as angina among those with CHD, and persistent cough and breathlessness among those with chronic bronchitis or emphysema, exert self-selection, especially if the work is physically demanding.

The healthy worker effect is strong for respiratory and cardiovascular diseases and weak for cancer.

For the reasons discussed, the SMR for all causes of death is difficult to interpret if it lies in the range of 80 to 100. However, the overall SMR is rather uninteresting in occupational epidemiology. Cause-specific SMR values are of more interest, especially if there is a prior hypothesis, according to which some specific exposure, some cocktail of exposures, or some other condition causes some specific disease. Rarely can one think of an occupational exposure that increases all causes of mortality, in contrast to social class, which has a strong influence on overall mortality.

The HWE hampers the interpretation of many cause-specific SMR values also. However, as far as cancer is concerned, the HWE does not make an occupational cohort study totally uninterpretable. One should especially compare the SMR values for specific sites, the hypothesized one being the most important. If the SMR for one site is high, but nearly normal for the others, the finding is an argument in favor of a true effect. However, the masking of true effects is a more serious problem, and therefore negative confounding, uncontrollable due to lack of information, often complicates the interpretation of the results. For this reason, the general population is not a good reference category even in cancer studies.

Example 15. Suppose a study shows a slightly elevated $\widehat{SMR}$ for lung cancer, say 132, in an occupational cohort of foundry workers. Is it due to some foundry exposure, such as silica dust or polycyclic aromatic hydrocarbons, or both, or to smoking? One may assume that foundry workers smoke much, and it may even be possible to get some proxy measure of the smoking by interviewing current workers, but because the smoking habits of the general population are not known well enough, the problem usually remains unsolved. (Of course, if the SMR is higher, say over 200, it cannot be explained by smoking alone; see Table 2.) One can get some hints from the $\widehat{SMR}$ values for other smoking-related diseases, such as bladder cancer, CHD, and emphysema. If these values are low, an occupational etiology becomes more credible and vice versa, but no firm conclusions can be drawn.

Although there are some methods by which the HWE can be reduced, however, none of them are completely satisfactory. One is not to start the computing of person-years before 5 to 10 years have elapsed from the beginning of employment. Furthermore, the analysis should focus separately on different calendar periods, different age categories, and different periods of follow-up. If exposure data or details of the employment history are available, it is important at least to dichotomize the exposed cohort into heavily and lightly exposed and to compare these subcohorts mutually. However, these refinements of analysis require large exposed cohorts, often much larger than those available for study.

In view of these considerations, one should avoid using the general population as a reference category whenever possible. It is true that good ad hoc reference groups may be hard to find and that using an ad hoc reference group doubles the costs of the study, both in terms of work and money, but that is the price one has to pay for quality. One valid, reliable, and efficient study is more informative than ten weak and uninterpretable ones. True, in order for statistical power to reach a sufficient level, the reference group must be rather large, and this too can be expensive. On the other hand, both exposure (meaning both other exposures and the absence of the exposure under study) and potential confounders can be measured from a statistical sample of the whole material, although the morbidity or mortality is recorded from the whole group. This is one way of decreasing costs.

Another method with which to avoid the HWE is to form the "exposed" cohort base according to liberal criteria for inclusion. Even unexposed subjects can be admitted. The analysis can then be made using a case-referent design within the cohort base. In such a design, all the cases of the disease and a sample of noncases, represented by another disease, or of the whole study base are compared with respect to the exposure of interest. The liberal inclusion criteria permit large enough exposure contrasts, and it becomes possible to study the effects of the exposure of interest without the use of the general population. However, a cohort defined in this way is not suitable for a conventional SMR analysis, because the inclusion of slightly exposed subjects dilutes the effect if the cohort is being analyzed as a homogeneous group (see Chapter 4).

PRECISION

Random errors result from the imprecision of single measurements. The point estimate of the summary result of the study (e.g., the $\widehat{RR}$) also has a random variation—the smaller the study, the larger the variation.

Imprecision occurs whenever the method of measurement is insensitive or its specificity is poor. Crude methods give rise to variation around the mean, and this variation cannot be adjusted by a correction factor or any other method. For example, the error of a nonspecific analytical method measuring a certain chemical, say, a metabolite of a toxic agent, may have a constant direction (e.g., always giving values that are too high because of its very nonspecificity). Because it also measures some other chemical, in contrast to a more specific method, one can never tell how much in error the result is. Many older methods for analyzing metabolites of xenobiotics in the urine resulted in values that were too high, but not constantly so, compared with the results of more modern and more specific methods (e.g., gas chromatography).

The difference between the nature of random errors and systematic errors is illustrated in Figure 5. Random errors level out, at least in large materials. (In technical terms they have a distribution whose mathematical mean value = 0.) They can be compared with poor target shooting, where the hits are spread around the bullseye. Even if there is no bullseye, the average of the hits may lie in the middle (Figure 5). In a shooting competition the result would be far from a gold medal. In a scientific study such a scatter gives rise to "background noise." Reaching statistical significance becomes difficult because the range of variation is one of the components of significance tests.

A systematic error is very different. It can be compared to a concentrated hit of the target, but in the wrong place (e.g., around score 2 at half past four o'clock in Figure 5). Such an error can be corrected if the aim of the rifle is adjusted properly—then the gold medal is within reach. In a scientific study one can, in the same manner of speaking, adjust for measuring errors, provided their magnitude is known, or correct for confounding (but not for selection bias). If the correction succeeds, the result becomes more accurate, although its point estimate varies randomly depending on the study size. The limits for such random variation can be estimated statistically in contrast to a systematic error, whose presence eliminates the assumptions for significance testing.

The random variation of the summary result, say, the estimate of the RR of the whole study, has already been referred to. In the following discussion of this random variation, it is assumed that systematic errors have been controlled.

The smaller the study, the more the estimate of the RR varies by chance. Suppose that a small study yields an $\widehat{RR}$ of 8 with a 95% confidence interval of 0.6--106. A repetition of the study could, by pure chance, yield any $\widehat{RR}$ within this range, and even outside it in extreme cases. Because the lower bound is less than 1, the result is not statistically significant, and the likelihood that $\widehat{RR} = 8$ indeed indicates excess risk is not convincing.

As the size of the study material increases, the confidence interval shrinks. In other words, the point estimate for the RR becomes more stable, and its random variation decreases. In a large material, the supposed $\widehat{RR}$ of 8 could have a 95% confidence interval of, say, 6.5--9.8, which is statistically highly significant; it strongly suggests that the increased risk is real. Even if the $\widehat{RR}$ were only 3, but the 95% confidence interval, say, 1.8--5.0, the result would be statistically significant, and more credible than the $\widehat{RR}$ of 8 in the small study.

The smaller the study, the greater the random variation of the rate ratio.

The term "statistically significant" was mentioned in respect to RR values having a lower confidence limit in excess of 1. There is, indeed, a connection

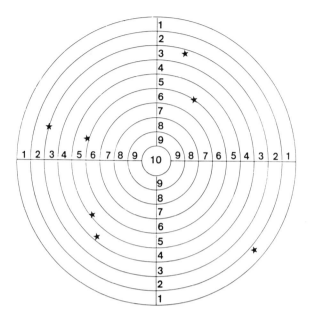

random error

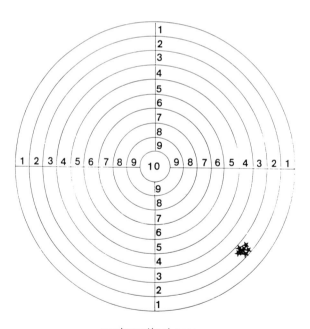

systematical error

Figures 5a and b. The difference between random and systematic errors can be compared with target shooting.

between the p-value and the lower confidence limit; in fact, one can say that they express the same thing in two different ways at the level of significance chosen. A statistical significance test gives a formal estimate of the probability of the observed difference between the study groups being ''true'' and not due to random variation. The issue is to test the *null hypothesis*, according to which there is no effect of the exposure on the particular outcome, against the unspecified alternative, the study hypothesis, according to which the exposure has an effect of a stated direction. The result of the statistical test gives an estimate of how frequently a difference of the magnitude observed can be expected to occur by pure chance in a study material of that size. There are several statistical tests by which this calculation can be made (depending on the study design and the distribution of the outcome variate), and from their result the p-value can be derived. The statistical test from which it is computed must fulfill certain model assumptions to be suitable for the study material in question. It is important to choose the correct statistic. The help of a skilled statistician (not only a personal computer) is needed for making the correct choice.

The p-value is a statistical concept familiar to most, but understood by few. It is characterized by that its small values support the correctness of the study hypothesis while large values support the null hypothesis, according to which the exposure in question has no effect. According to the classical definition, the p-value expresses the probability of obtaining results that are extreme or more extreme than the one observed by chance alone. A very low p-value indicates a low probability that the finding is due to chance and a high probability that it is due to a true effect of the exposure. Low p-values are uninformative, while high values support the correctness of the null hypothesis. However, the p-value conveys more information than that. It is a summary statistic which, in addition to the magnitude of the observed difference, takes into account the amount of information in the material (i.e., the size of the material, and how common the phenomenon of interest is in the material). In other words, the p-value expresses how probable the obtained result is under the null hypothesis, that is, the probability of achieving a difference such as the one found if no true difference exists, given the size of the material and the frequency of the phenomenon of interest in it. The interpretation of p-values is further discussed in Chapter 9.

The p-value is a partial summary of the evidence for or against the null hypothesis in the particular data.

Statistical significance is usually so defined that results yielding $p < 0.05$ are said to be significant. By definition then, one result out of 20 is statistically significant, even if no true effect existed. If p < 0.01 is chosen as the significance level, then one out of 100 results will be "significant" by definition. There can never be complete assurance that an observed result is not due to chance. The lower the p-value, the lower the probability, but it will never reach 100%.

The commonly used levels for statistical significance have no scientific foundation. There are no theoretical grounds for p = 0.04 being significant and for p = 0.06 being nonsignificant. This practice is not even based on a consensus from some expert group convened to penetrate this problem. Astonishingly enough, the cut-off points first adapted by experimenters and later mimicked by epidemiologists, are purely arbitrary. "Accepting" or "rejecting" hypotheses based on such arbitrary statistical cut-off points is not scientific in nature. A scientific conclusion can never be that mechanical and it should be based on true insight into the problem.

When planning a study, one conventionally defines a limit below which the null hypothesis will be rejected. This limit is called alpha. If the p-value obtained from the data is equal or lower than alpha, the results are considered to support the alternative hypothesis, and the null hypothesis is rejected. Usually the arbitrary limits of 0.05 or 0.01 are used for setting the alpha, with the inherent problems discussed earlier.

It is possible to compute formally the size of material needed to reach a statistically significant difference (delta) at each level of alpha. In other words, one can compute the probability of erroneously rejecting the null hypothesis, that is, of drawing a falsely positive conclusion when the true result is negative. This error is called *type I error* by statisticians. By choosing a low limit for alpha, the researcher reduces the possibility of that type of error, but the difference (delta) required or, alternatively, the size of the material becomes larger.

There is also another type of error, that of accepting the null hypothesis even if the study hypothesis was correct. In other words, one wrongly concludes that the exposure under study has no effect, even if it does have one in reality. Such approval can occur if the difference observed in a small material does not reach statistical significance. This phenomenon is called a *type II error* in statistical terms. Again, the problem arises from too mechanical an interpretation of p-values and a poor understanding of the limitations of statistical testing (see Chapter 9).

It has been the rule for researchers to concentrate on avoiding type I errors when deciding the sample size. However, type II errors should not be neglected, either, because a falsely negative conclusion can even be a more serious mistake than a falsely positive one. For example, falsely negative studies on carcinogenic agents can create a false feeling of safety and lead to neglect to carry out necessary hygienic improvements. Therefore, it is important to design a study so that the risk for type II errors is also minimized. The probability of avoiding type II errors is called the *power* of the study to detect true differences between the groups, and it is called 1-beta in statistical terms. It is also possible to compute the required study size for different levels of beta as a function of the RR, that is, how large should the material be in order for the researcher to be able to detect a certain risk with a sufficiently high probability (e.g., a power of 0.80). Formulas exist for computing both alpha and beta for different RR values. (See, e.g., References 6 and 34.)

However, some authorities are skeptical of such formal computations. According to Miettinen,[26] the first and foremost decision regarding the size of the study is whether the sample size should be zero or something else. He says that if it is not possible to design a study devoid of bias, zero is the only justifiable sample size. Otherwise one will only create confusion in addition to wasting money. Miettinen also says that it is difficult to define an optimal sample size with statistical methods. One cannot know in advance how big the found differences will be, the availability of the study material can be restricted, the funds are often limited, and, in research projects, unexpected events usually occur. In other words the optimal study size cannot be determined in advance statistically. However, even so, some advance formal and informal considerations will help planning the study. It may be prudent to begin the evaluation of what sample size is needed by first performing crude power calculations to obtain an approximation of how large a material is required for solving the problem. (Here one should be well aware of whether the objective is qualitative or quantitative.) Thereafter, the estimate should be refined informally by using the intuition of an experienced epidemiologist with good knowledge of the subject matter. If the outlook turns out doubtful, one should have courage enough to abandon the project.

GENERALIZATION

Generalization can mean the statistical generalization from a sample to a larger basic population, or it can mean the scientific generalization from one particular study experience to the abstract-general or to the level of scientific theories. In epidemiologic research, both types of generalization are made because the problems can be either particularistic or abstract.

A *particularistic* problem is bound to time and place, and therefore studies of such problems are descriptive only. The study material is then a sample drawn from a larger basic population. Examples of such problems are the level of lead exposure in different types of companies in a geographic area or the prevalence of hearing loss in shipyards. Such studies are done from statistically representative samples of, say, lead-using industries in a city or all shipyards in a country. In such a setting, the generalization is one of sample-to-population. Provided the samples are correctly chosen, that is, statistically representative, their results can be generalized to the larger base population.

Example 16. Suppose that 5% of randomly examined lead workers in Chicago have a blood lead level in excess of 60 μg/100 mL (approximately 3 μmol/L), and an additional 15% have values between 41 and 60 μg/dL. Suppose also that there are 14,000 exposed workers in this city. Then we can estimate that 700 workers are at risk of lead poisoning, and in all 2800 are in need of regular surveillance. However, generalizations hold only for that base population, and only for conditions prevailing at the time of the survey. The results cannot be generalized to another state or country, or to another time period. Their use is for administrative purposes.

The problems of generalization in *scientific research* are fundamentally different because in science the results of a study are being generalized beyond the data gathered from the particular study, and from the particular base population, to the sphere of abstract knowledge or "scientific truths." Now it is irrelevant how statistically representative the sample was of, say, all factories or of all workers in a country or in the whole world for that sake. Instead, the sample should represent a certain category of people, for example, male viscose rayon workers who have been exposed to carbon disulfide for at least 5 years. The purpose of scientific generalization is to determine if exposure to carbon disulfide in general causes or worsens CHD. For this problem it is totally irrelevant if the workers are representative of all Finnish men or if the plant is representative of all plants in the world. The generalization concerns whether carbon disulfide is cardiotoxic. If so, then exposure (of a certain intensity and duration) to this chemical is dangerous for everyone.

This is an example of the general, scientific conclusion which is the goal of scientific studies. Scientific interest may go even further. The generalization can be refined or rather specified to involve effect modifiers (i.e., to define factors that increase or diminish the cardiotoxic effects of carbon disulfide). In other words, does the increased risk occur only after a certain age, only in smokers, only among those with high blood lipids, does it persist after the cessation of exposure, and so forth? Such specification deepens the understanding of the mechanism of cardiotoxic action.

Scientific generalization goes from particular study results to an abstract-general level of knowledge.

Scientific inference relies much on the critical judgment of the researcher, and also on that of the reader of the study report. It is crucial to be able to place the new results into perspective while also taking into account existing knowledge (see Chapter 9). Generalization of results from a particular study requires that the study be valid. Generalizing biased results can only lead to wrong conclusions and confusion. Moreover, it is prudent not to draw too far–going conclusions from single epidemiologic studies because random errors, undetected bias or insensitivity may lead to wrong conclusions. Few single epidemiologic studies have been able to change prevailing scientific views fundamentally. Science usually advances by small steps, and knowledge must accumulate from several different sources in order to be able to create new theories.

REFERENCES

1. Ahlman, K., A.-L. Backman, and I. Hannunkari, et al. "Kivityöntekijöiden työolosuhteet ja terveydentila." in *Kansaneläkelaitoksen julkaisuja AL* No. 4 (Helsinki: Kansaneläkelaitos, 1975).
2. Ahlman, K., A.-L. Backman, R.-S. Koskela, and K. Luoma. "Satamatyöntekijöiden työolot ja terveydentila." in *Työterveyslaitoksen tutkimuksia* No. 105 (Helsinki: Työterveyslaitos, 1975).
3. Asp, S. "Confounding by variable smoking habits in different occupational groups," *Scand. J. Work Environ. Health* 10:325 (1984).
4. Axelson, O. "Aspects on confounding in occupational health epidemiology," *Scand. J. Work Environ. Health* 4:98 (1978).
5. Campbell, D. "Factors relevant to the validity of experiments in the social setting," *Psychol. Bull.* 54:297 (1957).
6. Feinstein, A. R. "Clinical biostatistics: XXXIV. The other side of 'statistical significance': alpha, beta, delta, and the calculation of sample size," *Clin. Pharmacol. Ther.* 18:491 (1975).
7. Fox, A. J., and P. F. Collier. "Low mortality rates in industrial cohort studies due to selection for work and survival in the industry," *Br. J. Prev. Soc. Med.* 30:225 (1976).
8. Greenland, S. "Modeling and variable selection in epidemiologic analysis," *Am. J. Public Health* 79:340 (1989).
9. Hansson, T. *Ländryggsbesvär och arbete.* (Stockholm: Arbetsmiljöfondens Rapporter, 1989.)
10. Hernberg, S., T. Kauppinen, R. Riala, M.-L. Korkala, and U. Asikainen. "Increased risk for primary liver cancer among women exposed to solvents," *Scand. J. Work Environ. Health* 14:356 (1988).
11. Hernberg, S., M.-L. Korkala, U. Asikainen, and R. Riala. "Primary liver cancer and exposure to solvents," *Int. Arch. Occup. Environ. Health* 54:147 (1984).
12. Hernberg, S., T. Partanen, C. H. Nordman, and P. Sumari. "Coronary heart disease among workers exposed to carbon disulphide," *Br. J. Ind. Med.* 27:313 (1970).
13. Hernberg, S., P. Westerholm, K. Schultz-Larsen, et al. "Nasal and sinonasal cancer: connection with occupational exposure in Denmark, Finland and Sweden," *Scand. J. Work Environ. Health* 9:315 (1983).
14. Industrial Disease Standards Panel. "Report to the Workers' Compensation Board on the Healthy Worker Effect," Industrial Diseases Standards Panel, Toronto, Ontario, 1988. (IDSP Rep. No 3.)
15. Kitagawa, E. M., and P. M. Hauser. *Differential Mortality in the United States* (Cambridge, MA: Harvard University Press, 1973).

16. Koskela, R. S., S. Hernberg, R. Kärävä, E. Järvinen, and M. Nurminen. "A mortality study of foundry workers," *Scand. J. Work Environ. Health* 2(Suppl. 1):73 (1976).

17. Koskela, R.-S., K. Luoma, and S. Hernberg. "Turnover and health selection among foundry workers," *Scand. J. Work Environ. Health* 2(Suppl. 1):90 (1976).

18. Kurppa, K., P. C. Holmberg, S. Hernberg, K. Rantala, R. Riala, and T. Nurminen. "Screening for occupational exposures and congenital malformations: preliminary results from a case-referent study," *Scand. J. Work Environ. Health* 9:89 (1983).

19. Lloyd, J. W., F. E. Lundin, C. K. Redmond, and P. B. Geiser. "Long-term mortality study of steelworkers: IV. Mortality by work area," *J. Occup. Med.* 12:151 (1970).

20. Mantel, N., and W. Haenszel. "Statistical aspects of the analysis of data from retrospective studies of disease," *J. Natl. Cancer Inst.* 22:719 (1959).

21. McMichael, A. J. "Standardized mortality ratios and the 'healthy worker effect': Scratching beneath the surface," *J. Occup. Med.* 18:165 (1976).

22. McMichael, A. J. "Assigning handicaps in the mortality stakes: an evaluation of the 'Healthy worker effect,' Report to the Workers' Compensation Board on the Healthy Worker Effect, Industrial Disease Standards Panel, Toronto, Ontario, 1988, p. 58 (IDSP Rep. No. 3.)

23. McMichael, A. J., R. Spirtas, and L. L. Kupper. "An epidemiologic study of mortality within a cohort of rubber workers 1964-72," *J. Occup. Med.* 16:458 (1974).

24. Meinhardt, T. J., R. J. Young, and R. W. Hartle. "Epidemiologic investigations of styrene-butadiene rubber production and reinforced plastics production," *Scand. J. Work Environ. Health* 4(Suppl. 2);240 (1978).

25. Miettinen, O. S. "Matching and design efficiency in retrospective studies," *Am. J. Epidemiol.* 91:111 (1970).

26. Miettinen, O. S. *Theoretical Epidemiology. Principles of Occurrence Research in Medicine* (New York: John Wiley & Sons, 1985).

27. Miettinen, O. S. "The healthy worker effect," Report to the Workers' Compensation Board on the Healthy Worker Effect. Industrial Disease Standards Panel, Toronto, Ontario, 1988, p. 72. (IDSP Rep. No. 3.)

28. Monson, R. R. "Healthy worker effect," Report to the Workers' Compensation Board on the Healthy Worker Effect. Industrial Disease Standards Panel, Toronto, Ontario, 1988, p. 77. (IDSP Rep. No. 3.)

29. Newhouse, M. L. "A study of the mortality of workers in an asbestos factory," *Br. J. Ind. Med.* 26:294 (1969).

30. Ott, M. G. "Determinants of mortality in an industrial population," *J. Occup. Med.* 18:171 (1976).

31. Pershagen, G., and O. Axelson. "A validation of questionnaire information on occupational exposure and smoking," *Scand. J. Work Environ. Health* 8:24 (1982).

32. Rothman, K. J. *Modern Epidemiology* (Boston, MA: Little Brown, 1986).

33. Sauli, H. *Occupational Mortality in 1971-75* (Helsinki: Central Statistical Office of Finland, 1979).

34. Schlesselman, J. J. *Case-Control Studies: Design, Conduct, Analysis* (Monographs in Epidemiology and Biostatistics), (New York: Oxford University Press, 1982).

35. Wang, J.-D., and O. S. Miettinen. "Occupational mortality studies: principles of validity," *Scand. J. Work Environ. Health* 8:153 (1982).

CHAPTER 6

Specific Problems in the Study of Some Work-Related Disorders*

INTRODUCTION

When a causal relation between an occupational exposure and a specific disease is clear, the disease is defined as occupational both medically and usually legally. However, work and work conditions may, in addition, contribute to the development of nonspecific morbidity, either through causation or aggravation, or even indirectly through the occupationally related life-style of the worker. Conceptually work-related diseases thus comprise a wide range of morbidity, related in some way or another—not necessarily causally—to occupation, work, or work conditions. Classical occupational diseases constitute one end of the continuum, while disorders with a very slight or uncertain occupational connection are at the other. Many of the diseases within the continuum may be work-related under certain conditions only, and their etiology is always multicausal.

According to the definition of the World Health Organization (WHO),[52] work-related diseases are multifactorial diseases for which occupation, work, or work conditions may be one of many etiologic factors. Classical occupational diseases are excluded from this concept according to WHO's definition. However, there are other definitions, among them that of the National Institute for Occupational Safety and Health (NIOSH), which include occupational diseases in the definition.

Occupational factors can also aggravate, accelerate or exacerbate diseases with nonoccupational origins. In this case, work is *related* to, although not *etiologic* for those conditions. Finally, work can have beneficial rehabilitative effects on certain pathological conditions, provided the workers concerned are properly placed in jobs suited to their capacities and limitations.[11]

Because it is possible to improve work conditions, work-related disorders are, at least in principle, preventable. However, before effective prevention can be accomplished, the problem must be identified and quantified. Epidemiologic research has an important role in this process. Work conditions vary from one situation to another; hence, the strength of the occupational etiological factor also varies. This variation can lead to seemingly discrepant results in different studies. In other words, in studies on the same disease, an occupational etiology can sometimes be identified, but not always. The

---

* This chapter is partly based on the author's working paper to the X Joint ILO/WHO Committee Meeting on "Epidemiology of Work-Related Diseases and Injuries."

same is true when the degree of work-relatedness is different in different settings. Therefore, not only identifying but also quantifying, the work-related etiologic fraction is important for efficient (especially cost-efficient) prevention of work-related disorders. This chapter addresses the problems inherent in epidemiologic research aimed at identifying and quantifying the work-related etiology of five major disease categories: cancer, chronic nonspecific respiratory disease, musculoskeletal disorders, coronary heart disease, and behavioral responses and psychosomatic symptoms.

In principle, the epidemiologic study of work-related diseases does not, in general, differ from epidemiologic research. It therefore suffers from the inherent difficulties of all nonexperimental research, for example, in providing evidence for or against the causality of an observed association between two phenomena. What is typical, however, is that the occupational etiologic fraction (see Chapter 4) of a work-related disease (not regarded as a classical occupational disease) is comparatively small. In other words, many nonoccupational causes also contribute to the etiology of the disease in question, and usually their shares, taken together, are greater than that of the occupational factor. This situation creates problems both for the design of epidemiologic studies and for the interpretation of their results.

The demonstration of a slight increase in the occurrence of a common disorder among persons exposed to a work-related factor requires a large study and a sharp design. The latter requirement means that random errors, such as sampling errors, nondifferential misclassifications, and other measurement errors, indeed must be kept to a minimum. The better the design, the smaller the work-related effects can be and still be demonstrated. However, in general, work-related etiologic fractions among the exposed of some 20% or less are very difficult or impossible to reveal by means of epidemiologic methods.

Interpretation and synthesis of results from different studies must take into account both variations in the validity and sensitivity of single studies and the fact that variations in exposure intensity between studies can account for seemingly inconsistent results. While the scientific community in general is alerted to look for biases, especially those creating a falsely positive effect, little attention has usually been paid to the identification of "false negativity," which is usually due to either small sample size, insensitivity of design, random error, nondifferential misclassification of exposure, or combinations of these circumstances (see Chapter 9). Interstudy variation with regard to exposure intensity and duration can create seeming inconsistency in study results especially if exposure data are weak. The reader should realize that exposure data of poor quality can mask even strong true effects. Not even ten "negative" studies ("negative" because of poor quality of exposure data) "contradict" one positive finding if the latter is based on sound data. Lacking or insufficient exposure data, and even worse, erroneous assumptions derived from weak data and served as facts in scientific articles, have indeed often created confusion and seeming conflict when the issue has been to identify and quantify occupational etiologic factors. Moreover, the genesis of multi-factorial diseases can indeed be complicated, and sometimes lacking knowledge on interactions between different "contributing causes" and on how "sufficient causes" are composed can also render it difficult to explain why an occupational factor can be demonstrated in some instances but not in others. For example, several studies in Europe have shown that exposure to carbon disulfide is associated with an excess rate of coronary heart disease, but this appears not to be the case in Japan.[44,45] Modifying effects of other coronary risk factors, whose occurrence is different in Europe and Japan (e.g., diet), may explain this puzzling difference.

While the qualitative aspect of the work-relatedness of a disease is abstract-general (scientific), the quantitative aspect is particularistic (bound to time and place). In other words, if one, for example, accepts the studies showing that exposure to carbon disulfide contributes to the causation of coronary heart disease, then this is a generally applicable biomedical fact. By contrast, the *strength* of this etiologic factor varies with time and place. It is greater when exposure levels are high, and it is perhaps modified by other risk factors, which vary among different populations, such as dietary fat intake and smoking (see Chapter 1).

CANCER

Occupational Exposures

Some cancers were recognized long ago as being associated with occupational exposures. The first observation was made by Sir Percival Pott, who, in 1775 noted a high occurrence of scrotal cancer among chimney sweeps. In 1895 Rehn reported three cases of urinary bladder cancer among 45 workers in an aniline dye factory. The cause was first mistakenly belived to be aniline, but subsequent studies in several other countries identified the causative agents as β-naphthylamine and benzidine. Since then, many occupational exposures have been identified as certain or probable carcinogens. Epidemiologic studies on occupational cancer are common today and provide increased evidence for the carcinogenic effects of occupational exposures.

Since 1969, the International Agency for Research on Cancer (IARC) has conducted a program to evaluate the carcinogenic risk of chemicals to humans. This program has resulted in the publication of evaluative monographs on a large number of individual chemicals or groups of chemicals. In mid 1990, 48 monograph volumes had been published. In 1987 an expert group updated volumes 1 to 42, and, as a result, IARC published its so-called Supplement 7, containing overall evaluations of the human carcinogenity of more than 700 chemicals, groups of chemicals, industrial processes, occupational exposures, and cultural habits.[17] The chemicals or, alternatively, exposure conditions were classified into:

Table 1. Occupational Carcinogens for Which the Evidence is Sufficient

Exposure	Main Target Organs
4-Aminobiphenyl	Bladder
Arsenic and certain arsenic compounds	Skin, lung
Asbestos	Lung, pleura, peritoneum
Benzene	Bone marrow
Benzidine	Bladder
Bis(chloromethyl)ether and technical-grade chloromethyl methyl ether	Lung
Chromium and certain chromium compounds	Lung
Coal tars	Skin
Coal-tar pitches	Skin
Mineral oils (certain)	Skin
Mustard gas	Respiratory tract
Naphthylamine	Bladder
Nickel and nickel compounds	Nasal, sinus, lung
Shaleoils	Skin
Soots	Skin, lung
Talc containing asbestiform fibers	Lung
Vinyl chloride	Liver

Source: Data from IARC[17] and Vainio.[47]

- Group 1:   Carcinogenic to humans

- Group 2A: Probably carcinogenic to humans

- Group 2B: Possibly carcinogenic to humans

- Group 3:   Not classifiable as to their carcinogenicity to humans

- Group 4:   Probably not carcinogenic to humans

In order for a chemical to become classified into group 1, "sufficient evidence" for carcinogenicity in humans is required. The IARC supplement[17] defines this as follows: "a causal relationship has been established between exposure to the agent and human cancer. That is, a positive relationship has been observed between exposure to the agent and cancer in studies in which chance, bias and confounding could be ruled out with reasonable confidence" (p. 30). For agents classified into group 2A, the requirement is "limited" evidence for humans and "sufficient" for experimental animals (see Reference 17).

No more than 17 occupationally used agents or mixtures could be classified into group 1 in 1987. They are listed in Table 1. In addition, 11 industrial processes were considered to be causally associated with human cancer (Table 2).

Considering the large number of agents for which there is animal evidence of carcinogenicity, it is, at first sight, astonishing that the list of established human carcinogens is so short. However, the problems inherent in epide-

Table 2. Industrial Processes Causally Associated with Cancer in Humans

Process	Main Target Organs
Aluminum production	Lung
Auramine manufacture	Bladder
Boot and shoe manufacture and repair	Bone marrow, nasal sinus
Coal gasification (older process)	Skin, lung
Coke production	Skin, lung
Furniture manufacture (hardwood dust)	Nasal, sinus
Isopropyl alcohol manufacture (strong acid process)	Nasal, sinus
Iron and steel founding	Lung
Manufacture of magenta	Bladder
Rubber industry	Bladder, bone marrow
Underground hematite mining (with exposure to radon)	Lung

Source: Data from IARC[17] and Vainio.

Table 3. Some Probable (2A) and Possible (2B) Human Carcinogens in Need of More Epidemiologic Studies

Agent (2A)	Agent (2B)
Acrylonitrile	Bitumens
Beryllium and compounds	Carbon tetrachloride
	Chlorophenols
Creosotes	Chlorophenoxy herbicides
Epichlorhydrin	Hexachlorobenzene
Ethylene oxide	Hydrazine
Formaldehyde	Styrene
Silica	Tetrachloroethylene

miologic studies of occupational cancer, such as mixed exposure patterns, small exposed populations, lack of available exposure data, and low exposure levels, can explain why so few agents have been proved to be human carcinogens. Furthermore, many chemicals that are animal carcinogens are used only under laboratory conditions, or perhaps in a few small plants, and therefore epidemiologic studies are impossible. Another important and all too frequent (but remediable) reason for the lack of conclusive data is that many studies have thus far been of poor quality. Studies that contain bias increase the prevailing confusion and add nothing to existing knowledge. The same can be said of insensitive studies resulting in falsely negative conclusions.

Another problem is that so many researchers tend to favor "fashion carcinogens." Instead of repeating expensive cohort studies all over again, for example, on asbestos, nickel, hardwood dust, and other established carcinogens, they should instead choose widely used agents for which conclusive evidence is lacking. A proposal for research priorities, compiled from IARC's categories 2A and 2B, is presented in Table 3.

IARC's group 3 also includes several agents that could and should be given more epidemiologic attention: carbon black, chlordane, lead, and trichloroethylene.

Although cancer epidemiology first and foremost tries to identify and quantify carcinogenic risks, not to explain their mechanisms, it is useful to bear in mind also that carcinogenesis is a multistage process. It is common to speak about "initiators," which set the carcinogenic process in motion mainly by causing DNA damage, and "promotors," which provide the final stimulus for the neoplastic process. However, while some agents act at different stages of the multistage process, most identified carcinogens are "complete," that is, they have both initiating and promoting activities.[47] Action at different stages helps explain the synergistic effects between two carcinogens that have sometimes been observed, for example, between asbestos exposure and smoking. In the epidemiologic study of occupational cancer, the multistage process calls for thorough analysis of time relations between exposure and outcome. If a simplification is permitted, one could say that initiators have a long latency period, while promotors have a short one. However, complete carcinogens may act as initators at low doses and as promotors at high doses, so the problem can, indeed, be more complicated. Furthermore, because humans are usually exposed to a multitude of agents, complicated interactive patterns may confuse the time relation, especially since enough detailed exposure data are usually lacking. "Cocktail exposures," especially whenever many chemicals are involved at comparatively low exposure intensities, are becoming more and more common in today's "chemicalized" world, and their effects may elude any epidemiologic evaluation.

Levels of Cancer Epidemiology

The work-relatedness of cancer can be studied epidemiologically by means of several different approaches. The crudest level is to relate morbidity data in a cancer register to occupational categories. This is not an efficient method for the reasons discussed in Chapter 3. Somewhat better information can be gained if cancer register data are linked to occupations reported in earlier censuses, say, 10 or 20 years earlier. Cancer data can also be linked to other registers containing direct or indirect exposure data, such as registers of occupational diseases or employment records. But this type of information is suggestive at most, and misclassifications of exposure tend to mask true risks.

Register linkage epidemiology has recently been improved in Sweden. There a register, "Miljödataregistret" has supplemented occupational titles with the name of the workplace and the domicile of the person. Linking the occupational data of the 1960 census to cancer incidence data of, say, the 1980s can produce more accurate information about the work-relatedness of various cancer forms than conventional linkage practices.

Example 1. A recently published study[30] can be considered an attempt to test the sensitivity of that approach. Mesothelioma, which has a known connection with a number of asbestos-exposed occupations, was chosen as the "test cancer." The aim was to determine how well this type of linkage could detect occupations previously known to cause mesothelioma. The results were promising. Although one-digit (very broad) occupational codes gave no useful information, two-digit codes gave suggestive results and three-digit codes recognized most occupations known to entail exposure to asbestos. Typical branches of industry (shipbuilding, construction of railroad engines, insulation) all gave rate ratios ranging from 3 to 7. However, also less well-recognized occupational categories showed increased risk for mesothelioma, for example, sugar plant workers (SIR 6.3) and pulp and paper workers (SIR 4.7). If the later results can be confirmed in more specific studies, they indicate previous, perhaps unrecognized, use of asbestos in these industries, for example, in the insulation of sugar boilers or as the occurrence of asbestos in the form of impurities in the talc used for paper production.

This example illustrates that at least suggestive evidence of high cancer risk can be obtained from good registers provided the conventional register data on occupation are made more specific. It is however doubtful that medium and lower risks can be detected with this methodology. The same can be said whenever only a minor part of those falling into an occupational category are exposed to carcinogens, even if their exposure were of high intensity. Work-related cancer can also be investigated by means of proportionate mortality studies, which can provide the first signals of increased cancer risk. The weaknesses of PMR studies have been discussed in Chapter 4.

The cohort approach is perhaps the most traditional design for studying occupational cancer. Its advantage is the possibility to include several cancers at a time, and its disadvantage lies in the huge amount of work involved. Unfortunately, most cohort studies on occupational cancer have used the general population as the reference category. This practice has created much confusion because of the healthy worker effect and other types of comparison bias (see Chapters 5 and 9). During the last decade or so, a case-referent analysis of a cohort base has emerged and has provided a useful complement to the classical cohort design. Provided exposure contrasts are sufficiently large, and provided enough detailed exposure data can be found retrospectively, this approach overcomes most of the validity problems arising from the use of the general population as the reference category. A case-referent design drawing cases and referents from a dynamic population base often provides a good alternative to the use of a cohort base. Because the dynamic population base is often very large, sometimes the population-time experience of a whole country, rare forms of cancer can also be studied. National or regional cancer registers are best suited for this approach; hospital or parish registers are also possible sources for cases and referents. Problems arise whenever the exposure of interest is rare or ill defined. Recall bias must also be considered (see Chapter 5). To overcome this last mentioned problem, at least partly, patients with some other cancer form, unrelated to the exposure(s) under study, are often used as referents. Cancer referents can also be drawn as a sample from a cancer register.

Problems in Study Design

The long latency period between the start of exposure and the manifestation of the disease is perhaps the single factor that causes the worst problem for the epidemiologic study of work-related causes for cancer. Sometimes the mean latency time is as long as 30 to 40 years, as, for example, shown for asbestos-induced mesothelioma. Other cancer types may have shorter latency periods, but even so there is a lag of many years, even decades, between initiation and manifestation. It is believed that initiators that cause genetic damage to DNA usually have long latency periods, while promotors exerting their action in the final stages of carcinogenesis have short latencies. Complete carcinogens exert their action in several steps, complicating the study of time relations. For example, cigarette smoke is both an initiator and a promotor, and this fact is quite plausible considering the complex composition of cigarette smoke. In addition, both the length of the latency time and the magnitude of the excess risk may vary depending on, among other things, the age of the person when the exposure began, the duration and strength of the exposure, and other concomitant chemical exposures. The heterogeneity caused by these and other factors tends to lower the sensitivity of epidemiologic cancer studies.

The long latency period observed for many carcinogens has the practical consequence that epidemiologic cancer studies must usually be retrospectively timed. The worst disadvantage of retrospective timing is that the quality of exposure data and other important information suffers. Quantitative (dose-response) studies especially become difficult or impossible to carry out whenever exposure data are poor.

The long latency period also means that epidemiologic methods cannot be relied upon for the detection of new carcinogens, because newly introduced chemicals would then be dispersed in the occupational and even the general environment for some decades before being classified as carcinogens. Hence the requirement of epidemiologic evidence as the ''final'' proof of the carcinogenicity of some chemical has severe disadvantages. Regulatory and other preventive action must be taken on the basis of experimental evidence, even if the ''final'' proof is not yet available. Consequently, from a regulatory point of view, many countries consider the chemicals listed in IARC's category 2A and even some chemicals in 2B as proved carcinogens.

However, although the classification of new chemicals must be based on experimental methods, epidemiologic studies on currently used chemicals that are considered as probable or possible human carcinogens, and, of course, also on currently unclassifiable chemicals, are highly recommendable when-ever feasible.

Epidemiologic methods are insensitive and slow. The first de-tection of the carcinogenic properties of a chemical must, there-fore, rely on experimental methods.

The turnover of workers is another problem that is partially connected with the long time lag between first exposure and the manifestation of cancer. High turnover complicates the tracing of those who have changed employment or retired. This is especially a problem in countries having poor population registers, or whenever confidentiality legislation restricts the use of such registers. In Denmark, Finland, Norway, and Sweden, all having excellent population registers, one can usually trace 97 to 99% of the original cohort members, sometimes even all of them, but it is a laborious task. In many other countries, where tracing has to be carried out through the interviewing of close relatives or work colleagues or through the peruse of telephone directories, credit card registers and the like, 90% may be the best that can be achieved. The less success, the greater the likelihood for bias, because untraceable individuals probably differ from traceable ones. One should, therefore, exert every effort to achieve tracing that is as complete as possible. The requirement of a few years of minimum exposure time as an eligibility criterion reduces the tracing effort because turnover is always much higher during the first year of employment than later on.

High turnover results in short exposure times for a large propor-tion of the cohort. In addition, it increases the costs of tracing dropouts.

Turnover also results in a large proportion of the originally enlisted cohort accruing short exposure times. In qualitative research the most valuable in-formation comes from the study of individuals with long-term exposure to high intensities. Even a seemingly large cohort may contain few individuals fulfilling this criterion if turnover is high. This is yet another circumstance that lowers the sensitivity of epidemiologic cancer studies. However, in quan-titative research, exposure heterogeneity is useful, but then the number of person-years in each subcategory of exposure must be large enough.

However, whenever the problem is qualitative and the researcher succumbs to the temptation to include workers with short and low exposure into the cohort to increase its size, "dilution" of the effect results. In many workplaces several so-called "exposed" workers are not truly exposed. As long as the cohort is to be analyzed as a homogeneous group, inclusion of misclassified "exposed" workers strongly dilutes the effect.

The situation is different, however, if the data are to be analyzed by a case-referent approach. Then exposure contrasts become a resource, and it is even advantageous to include unexposed individuals in the study base. The case-referent approach, of course, cannot do away with problems arising from too few heavily exposed individuals (e.g., resulting in few "exposed" cases). However, because so much less work is involved than with a census approach, increasing the size of the study base, for example, by enrolling more similar companies, becomes a workable alternative. Of course the key question is, as in all cancer studies, to secure accurate and detailed exposure data. An experienced hygienist is needed for this purpose. Even so, retrospective exposure data may be unreliable, and misclassifications are likely to occur. Concurrent or consecutive occupational exposure to several chemicals, together with nonoccupational exposures, also complicate the study design and the interpretation of the results. Most workers have such exposure patterns, and, because the time period of interest is long, the chances of sorting out complex exposure patterns are not good. Again, a case-referent design has more potential than a census type of study because more effort can be devoted to elucidating the exposure of the sample when an entire base population need not be involved.

Mixed exposure patterns are a common problem in cancer epidemiology.

The problems discussed so far are difficult or impossible to overcome because they are inherent in the nature of the problem. For example, the long latency time is a characteristic of occupational cancer and cannot therefore be avoided. Likewise, a study may have to be abandoned because there are no possibilities to solve questions like missing exposure data or high turnover. On the other hand, sometimes it is really possible to find populations for which the effects of these problems are less, for example, workers employed by large companies with low turnover, good past exposure records, and few simultaneously occurring exposures. Such opportunities should not be missed.

Some other types of problems are more specific to time and place. They may then create insurmountable problems under certain circumstances, while their effect can be overcome in others. Problems arising from poor or missing exposure data have already been mentioned. Although problems in securing past exposure data occur in almost every cancer study, there are indeed workplaces with satisfactory records; sometimes even hygienic measurements are available. Such opportunities should be utilized because one good study can provide more conclusive data than many weaker studies combined. In addition, data on potential confounders (e.g., smoking) may or may not be available. If the researcher has several options for study material, those with available data on exposures and potential confounders should, of course, be preferred. If the data are poor, it may be best to abandon that potential study.

Misclassification can also arise from misdiagnoses of the cancer. In countries having good cancer registers, the problem is usually one of differentiating between primary and metastatic cancer, or between different histological subtypes. Cancers of the elderly, in particular, may be misclassified because autopsies are not performed as frequently as for younger persons. In countries with less accurate cancer registration the error may, of course, be worse.

Example 2. In a Finnish case-referent study on primary liver cancer, 182 cases were found in the cancer register during a 2-year period. Of them, 16 could not be confirmed as primary liver cancer by the team's pathologist. Another 28 diagnoses were based on clinical data alone. The most common sources of misclassification were metastatic tumors and invasive growth from neighboring organs. However, the case series in this study was composed of incident cases which had not yet been checked by the register's pathologist. A subsequent study on earlier cases (that had been checked by the register) had fewer misclassifications but still a similar proportion of pathologically unverified diagnoses.

In case-referent studies misclassified diagnoses also dilute true effects. Whenever the exposure of interest really has a carcinogenic effect, it is clear that mistakenly including other cancers without any relation to the exposure, will lower the odds ratio. Therefore one should always ensure that the case diagnosis is correct in a case-referent study. However, as already pointed out in Chapter 5, if a cohort study employs the general population as the reference, the diagnoses of the exposed cohort should *not* be corrected because the reference category cannot be checked; this would result in information that is asymmetrical in quality (i.e., bias).

In a case-referent study, the cases' diagnoses should be as accurate as possible.

The use of the general population as a reference population is, although very common, not recommended. True, the healthy worker effect is smaller for cancers than for many other diseases, but, even so, the general population does not fulfill even the most fundamental criteria for comparison validity (as discussed in Chapters 5 and 9). Major confounding may arise from differences in social class structure between the cohort and the general population. Such confounding is likely to be positive when blue-collar cohorts are studied, but it is negative when white-collar categories, such as physicians, are concerned.

> *Example 3.* A study conducted by the Finnish Cancer Register revealed differences in the incidence of lung cancer between different occupational categories characterized by different social class structure.[40] The $\widehat{SMR}$ varied from 18 (religious work) to 208 (mining) for men aged 35 to 69 years during the study period 1975 to 1979, when the SMR for the whole male population was set at 100.

This example underscores how important it is to have a valid reference group, one comparable to the exposed group in all relevant respects except exposure. However, it must be admitted that such groups are not easily available. A case-referent design utilizing a large study base would provide an alternative to the cohort design, and it would help solve the comparability problems.

Recall bias is probably the most difficult validity problem of the case-referent approach (see Chapter 5). The use of alternative sources of information (exposure data from workplace sources, use of hygienic expertise) helps overcome this type of bias.

Except for the recall bias and sometimes confounding, most errors inherent in epidemiologic studies of occupational cancer have a negative, that is, an *effect-masking direction.* The sensitivity of epidemiologic studies to detect true risks is therefore rather low, especially for the cohort design. Therefore, one should always consider "negative" cohort studies with caution, especially whenever there is prior reason to suspect that a chemical is a carcinogen (e.g., experimental evidence). Epidemiologic methods are so crude that they can detect only strong or medium cancer risks, and, even then, decades of exposure must have passed from the onset of exposure.

Most of the errors inherent in epidemiologic studies of occupational cancer have a negative direction.

CHRONIC NONSPECIFIC RESPIRATORY DISEASE

Definition

The WHO expert committee on the identification and control of work-related diseases[52] stated that chronic non-specific respiratory disease (CNRD) is a general term used to describe the groups of conditions in which there is chronic sputum production and/or shortness of breath at rest and/or during exercise. These conditions include chronic bronchitis, emphysema, and bronchial asthma. All of these diseases may be acutely or chronically exacerbated and complicated by respiratory infections. Immunological mechanisms may be involved in some of them. They are undoubtedly diseases of multiple etiology and represent a classical example of disorders that may mainly be occupational in origin or partly work-related, as well as related to the social phenomena of urbanization and industrialization (p. 25).

The Committee drew attention to the fact that the same dust (e.g., cotton dust) can cause both a classical occupational disease (byssinosis) and CNRD. Another respiratory disease, asthma, when caused by a certain agent, may be compensated as an occupational disease in one country but not in another. In the same manner, bronchitis is compensated as "occupational" in some countries, but not in all. "Occupational" is a legal rather than medical concept in such cases.

Work-Related Risk Factors

Several risk factors are important in the etiology and pathogenesis of CNRD; among them are smoking, air pollution, weather, socioeconomic factors, familial and genetic factors, atopic predisposition (for asthma), bronchial reactivity, childhood respiratory disease, and occupational exposures. The many factors involved often complicate identification of the occupational relationship; however, there are many occupational groups for which the work-related etiologic fraction is substantial.

Occupations with an elevated prevalence of chronic bronchitis include coal and other miners, steel workers, foundry workers, pulp mill workers, bakers, farmers, and cotton workers.[52] In many developing countries, exposure to dusts from such plants as cotton, flax, hemp, grain, and wood is an important factor in the high occurrence of chronic bronchitis. Smoking is often an important cofactor; in some studies the effect of dust is evident in smokers only. Welders have also been studied extensively. The results have been conflicting, probably due to the variety of welding techniques, exposure intensities, and smoking habits in the different studies.[22,43]

Work-related bronchial asthma, a disorder with generalized obstruction of the airways, is caused by the inhalation of substances or materials that a worker manufactures or uses directly or those that are incidentally present at the worksite.[34] There are numerous known causes for work-related asthma, including exposure to metals, plastics, organic chemicals, pharmaceuticals, plant products, and animals. Generally speaking, the prevalence of work-related asthma is unknown.[7] However, there are data from some industries which show that about 5% of isocyanate workers develop asthma (NIOSH 1978).[37] Asthma has ranged between 10 and 45% among workers exposed to proteolytic enzymes and between 2 and 40% among workers exposed to grain dusts.[6] The prevalence of laboratory animal allergy among animal handlers varied between 15 and 30% and that of asthma between 2 and 12% in seven studies of a total of 2075 persons.[38] However, most of the available experience on work-related asthma has been derived from clinical materials and case reports, not from epidemiologic studies.

Indicators of Morbidity and Their Measurement

Although about 3% of all deaths, reported from 88 countries, were due to CNRD,[53] mortality is too crude an indicator for the study of work-related CNRD. In countries having morbidity registers, disability due to CNRD can be studied. Chronic disability gives a better estimate of its occurrence than mortality figures. One could, for example, form exposure-based cohorts (e.g., foundry workers, cotton workers), use personal identification numbers for identification, and then identify, from the register, those on disability pension and compare the result with that of the general population or a more valid reference group. In some countries (e.g., Finland), one can also obtain data on cause-specific sick leaves and free medication, which is provided for a number of chronic diseases, among them asthma. However, effective control of confounding requires more information than that available from large registers. Ad hoc studies are, therefore, better. In such studies, additional data (e.g., on smoking, infections, and concurrent exposures) can and should be collected from the study groups by means of questionnaires or interviews.

While confounding, in principle, can be controlled, health-based selection out of the exposed jobs is a more difficult problem even in studies with a longitudinal design. Although the rate of turnover can be assessed in a longitudinal design, those who remain in the job, and consequently acquire the most exposure, represent a "survivor population" whose primary health state and resistance to the exposure is above average.

A population-based case-referent study is sometimes an alternative to a cohort study. Cases of asthma (or CNRD, which however is more difficult to define) are compared to a sample of noncases, or a sample of the source population, with regard to past working history. This approach enables the researcher to find new causes of work-related lung disease, because, using the case-referent design, one can study many different exposures at a time. Similar studies could be designed for diffuse roentgenological fibrosis, impaired lung function (according to preset criteria), and some other conditions for which an occupational etiology would be plausible as a contributing factor.

However, in most instances, knowledge of the work-relatedness of CNRD and asthma is based on cross-sectional epidemiologic studies (or clinical observations). The indicators of respiratory disease have usually been questionnaires (or interviews), lung function tests, radiographic examinations, and, in some instances, immunologic tests. All these methods pose problems.

Questionnaires and interviews must be well validated to be reliable. Both their specificity and sensitivity should be known.

Example 4. The British Medical Research Council's bronchitis form, which has gained wide use in epidemiologic studies, was originally well validated. However, few researchers realize that this form was validated as an interview, not as a self-administered questionnaire. It was also validated in a country with an exceptionally high prevalence of chronic bronchitis. Furthermore, the original form was in English, but it has later been translated into several other languages. All these circumstances have changed the original situation so that it is questionable whether a translated version, used as a self-administered questionnaire in, say, a Scandinavian country with a low prevalence of bronchitis fulfills the criteria for validation.

Whenever lung function tests are used, it is important to keep in mind exactly what they measure. Little information can be gained from tests measuring obstruction in the greater airways (forced expiratory volume, forced vital capacity, etc.) when the condition under study is mainly a restrictive disorder (e.g., fibrosis). In such instances, emphasis should be placed on tests measuring diffusion, even though they may be more complicated to use in field studies. Successful measurement of lung function requires simple, repeatable tests. Cooperation of the subject is crucial. There may also be great interobserver variability, and the same technician should therefore, ideally, perform all the tests. If the use of only one technician is not feasible (e.g., too large a study material), the interobserver error must be measured and each of the technicians should examine the same proportion of exposed and reference subjects, even the same proportion of different subcategories of the exposed group. Otherwise an asymmetrical inaccuracy of observations easily results—one which distorts the true result of the study.

The use of radiological examinations is also complicated by inter- and intraobserver errors. Without being perfect, the most recent classification of the International Labour Office (ILO)[18] is the best method available for the radiographic estimation of fibrosis; hence, it should be employed whenever possible. There should be several readers who should be blinded with regard to both the exposure status of the subject and the time sequence of serial pictures. The inter- and intraobserver errors should be measured and reported.

The diagnosis of asthma is usually rather straightforward in hospitals, but in the epidemiologic setting the same thoroughness of examination is rarely possible, at least not in large populations. It is important to define strict criteria for a positive epidemiologic diagnosis of asthma. These criteria should be applied in a similar way to both the exposed and the reference groups, which thus should undergo the same examinations. A careful history is essential, which can be obtained either with a standardized questionnaire or a structured interview. Even so, the epidemiologic diagnosis of asthma is uncertain. One of the better questions, especially when the history taking spans many years, is plainly "Has a doctor ever said that you have asthma?" One should also remember that there are different patterns of reactions, namely, immediate, nonimmediate or late, as well as combined patterns. The immediate reactions occur within 15 to 30 minutes after exposure and are of relatively short duration. The nonimmediate or late reactions may (1) begin about 1 h after exposure and last for 2 to 3 h; (2) begin after 4 to 5 h and last for about 24 to 36 h, or (3) begin early in the morning during several days and subside during the day.[39] The possibility that any of these different patterns may occur must be accounted for in the standardized history-taking. Asthma may often be of the hyperreactive type, which means that, for example, cold or irritant gases can provoke attacks nonspecifically without an allergic mechanism being involved.

Other allergic manifestations (rhinitis, atopic symptoms) should also be included in the history. In addition, the evaluation of the results of lung function tests should take into consideration the fact that there are different patterns of reaction. A standardized histamine or metacholine provocation can be used as a nonspecific test to study hyperreactivity of the airways. A specific provocation test gives an even better confirmation of the diagnosis but is usually too complicated for field use. In some instances, the diagnosis may be difficult because airway obstruction can persist with no change in symptoms over weekends or vacations, or even after a person leaves the job. Asthma caused by small-molecular chemicals such as diisocyanates may cause persistent symptoms, which probably can be either of an immunologic or nonimmunologic origin or both.[24]

Other tests that can be used in epidemiologic surveys include skin testing, counting of eosinophilic granulocytes in blood or sputum, and seroimmunologic tests. It is important to test allergenic extracts before their epidemiologic use in order to exclude nonspecific irritant reactions. The use of positive and negative control tests is commendable. Seroimmunologic tests are useful but far more expensive than skin tests.

Assessment of Exposure

Whenever the study design is exposure-based, as in cohort studies and exposure-based cross sections of the study base, it is assumed that the exposure of interest is known in qualitative terms. For example, if the issue is bronchitis among coal miners, the cohort is formed according to exposure to coal dust, and, if it is asthma among mink farmers, exposure is supposed to be fur dust or excreta from minks. However, when broader exposure categories are studied (e.g., welders or foundry workers), a more-detailed characterization of the exposure is necessary. For example, there are many different welding methods, and these methods produce fumes with different chemical compositions, particle sizes, and other characteristics. In such situations, a proper characterization of the exposure composition is necessary for identifying the specific conditions causative of, say, the bronchitis. Failure to define the exposure probably accounts for at least part of the confusion now occurring in the literature on respiratory symptoms among welders. Exposure intensities should also be measured, especially when the study aims at establishing exposure-response relationships and the definition of a nonadverse-effect level.

Concomitant other exposures should also be identified and, if possible, quantified because they can modify the effects of the agent under study or they can be confounders if they are asymmetrically distributed across the study groups. For example, certain categories of foundry workers are exposed to the irritative agents formaldehyde and furans, in addition to sand dust and soot. It is, therefore, important to define exactly who is or has been exposed to what, and how much, when the bronchitis-causing effects of foundry dust are being assessed.

In studies of work-related asthma, the causative allergen should be identified in the work environment. Sometimes identification is straightforward, for example, in bakeries, but sometimes the exposure is mixed. Often impurities and by-products may be the causative agents—these then have to be identified. This can be a difficult task. Quantitative aspects are less important for allergic diseases than for CNRD, but, for some chemicals causing asthma, at least a crude exposure–response relationship exists, and hyperreactivity is also dose-dependent.

Smoking

Studies on work-related respiratory disorders can rarely be valid if smoking is not accounted for. Usually the smoking habits are not known prior to the study, or existing data are crude or unreliable. Detailed data on past and current smoking must therefore be collected by interview or questionnaire as a part of the study protocol. When the study is being designed, the contrasts between subcategories of smoking should be made great enough. For example, it may be cost-efficient to focus on heavy smokers and nonsmokers and exclude moderate smokers and ex-smokers from the study. Often the most pertinent information comes from comparisons between exposed and unexposed heavy smokers because the exposure in question and smoking may act synergistically. In other instances, the effect of smoking upon some parameter (e.g., the closing volume) may be so overwhelming that a work-related weaker etiologic factor cannot be identified. Comparisons between nonsmokers may yield the most relevant information.

How to classify ex-smokers often poses a problem. Sometimes they can be classified as nonsmokers (provided some time, 1 or 2 years, has elapsed), for example, when bronchitis is the issue. However, other effects of smoking are more irreversible (e.g., emphysema). Often some health-related cause may have been the reason why a person quit smoking, and then strong "effects" can be found among present nonsmokers. If the study material is sufficiently large, ex-smokers should perhaps be omitted completely. In some studies it may be necessary to also account for passive smoking. Passive smoking may be a work-related cause of CNRD, or it may act as a potential confounder in the study of other causes.

Other Validity Aspects

Many occupational exposures affecting the respiratory system cause distinct subjective symptoms which result in a marked health-based selection out of the job, the remaining workers representing a "survivor population." That such selection indeed occurs has been intuitive knowledge among practitioners for many years; some scientific studies have also documented this as fact. Workers with allergy and chronic obstructive lung disease tend to leave exposed jobs (e.g., Reference 10). Furthermore, plant physicians have long been restrictive in permitting atopics or those with chronic obstructive lung disease to take an "exposed" job. Hence any cross-sectional study of work-related lung diseases tends to underestimate the true effect of work.

Longitudinal studies may also suffer from selection bias. Preplacement examinations, if successful, result in a healthier-than-normal exposed group, and selective turnover out of the job leads to reduced exposure times for those who are the most affected by subjective symptoms. In many study protocols, a minimum exposure time is used as an eligibility criterion in order to increase the effectiveness of the investigation. If so, those having quit the job early will not become classified as exposed at all. Later dropouts who comply with the minimum exposure criteria create another type of problem. It is true that they can be found if tracing is successful, but they will have experienced less exposure than the "survivor population" and, for that matter, may even have recovered from their work-related disorder. This possibility, if not controlled for, severely distorts the quantitative assessment of the etiologic fraction.

Securing a valid baseline measurement for longitudinal studies is another difficult problem. Usually researchers start with a cross section of currently employed workers who, as already mentioned, respresent a "survivor population," but who nonetheless already may have some decrement of function as compared with their own (unknown) values before the exposure commenced. The ideal method would be to use a preemployment examination as the baseline, but that examination would require better than usual standardization and quality control of the routine lung function tests used. An ad hoc program for measuring preexposure values would be even better. Serial examinations combined with the tracing of dropouts (at least the reason for quitting should be recorded) would then give more reliable data than the commonly used approach.

MUSCULOSKELETAL DISORDERS

Low-Back Pain

Low-back pain is a symptom, not a disease entity. It has a multifactorial etiology, and occurs commonly in the entire population, in all age groups, in all social strata, and in all occupations. In the United States, musculoskeletal disorders are the leading cause of disability of working-age population, afflicting 19 million persons each year.[3] Back problems are a significant part of this group. The symptom of pain has many causes; it can result from inflammatory, degenerative, neoplastic, traumatic, and even psychogenic causes. Back problems are more common in heavy than in light work. Accidents and repeated microtraumas are important causes of low-back disorders. Young, unskilled, and inexperienced workers have a higher incidence of injuries than older, skilled, and experienced workers.[46] Stooping, sitting, and lifting, especially unexpectedly heavy loads, are also factors that contribute to back pain. Whole-body vibration (e.g., tractor or truck driving) is another probable cause.[46] The following occupational factors have been considered to cause or aggravate work-related low-back disorders:

- Injuries
- Work with frequent twisting and bending
- Work with much lifting, especially unexpected heavy loads, and/or other types of physically heavy handling of materials
- Heavy physical work
- Work involving static load
- Sitting work positions with concomitant exposure to whole-body vibration
- Psychosocial problems

However, sedentary work and physical inactivity have also been incriminated as being related to low-back pain. Human biological factors, such as physical size, strength, fitness, range of motion, work endurance, and the integrity of the musculoskeletal system play a role; back pain can result because of a discrepancy between the worker's capabilities and the work demands.[3] Recent prospective studies have shown that psychological and psychosocial factors are important causes of back-related sickness absenteeism.[4] Negative factors such as monotony, poor social relations, poor job satisfaction, and a low level of education have been associated with high sickness absence due to back problems.[14] This complex picture renders the epidemiologic study of low-back pain extremely difficult.

Neck and Upper-Limb Disorders

Neck and upper-limb disorders represent a variety of conditions, some of them ill defined. Among these are cervical spondylosis, cervical disc disease, the thoracic outlet syndrome, the tension neck syndrome, shoulder joint osteoarthrosis, rotator cuff tendinitis, tenosynovitis, peritendinitis, and epicondylitis. All these syndromes have multiple causes, and, in addition, several predisposing factors increase the chances of pain developing. Among the causes for shoulder and neck pain are inflammatory reactions in the synovial membrane and bursa system, as well as degenerative disorders of the cartilage, ligaments, and tendons. In addition, muscular, vascular, and neurological disorders may cause shoulder pain, and there may be referred pain from the chest organs.

A meta-analysis of the literature on shoulder–neck diseases in different occupational groups has shown some connections with poor work conditions or postures.[13] Working with the hands at shoulder level was associated with rotator cuff tendinitis, tasks with repetitive arm movements with the thoracic outlet syndrome, and keyboard operating with the tension neck syndrome. The prevalence of the cervical syndrome was high among slaughterhouse workers, scissor makers, and civil servants, as compared with various reference groups. Assembly-line packers had a high prevalence of the thoracic outlet syndrome, whereas shipyard welders, plate workers, and industrial workers working above shoulder height had a high prevalence of rotator cuff tendinitis. The tension neck syndrome was prevalent in many occupations, especially in film rollers. The importance of precipitating injury has also been considered, but the studies are not quite conclusive.[2]

Peritendinitis and tenosynovitis are often due to overexertion or a change in daily routine, such as the resumption of new tasks on return from a leave of absence. In addition, blunt trauma and sprain can cause these symptoms. Epicondylitis, or the tennis elbow syndrome, is usually triggered by exertion of the finger and wrist extensors.[28] Repetitive manual tasks have been incriminated as causing the tennis elbow syndrome, but there is little if any valid research supporting this assumption.[48]

Osteoarthrosis

Osteoarthrosis is a common cause of impairment, although it is underrecorded in morbidity statistics.[2] This lack may at least partly be due to diagnostic confusion. Arthrosis can be defined as radiographically demonstrable osteophytes in a joint; however, most individuals over 50 years of age have this finding and are symptom-free nevertheless.

Osteoarthrosis is a disease of the elderly. Apart from age, obesity, heredity, and occupational strain are also risk factors. Frequent heavy lifting, work in awkward postures, vibration, repetitive strain, and heavy work in general appear to be work-related causes of osteoarthrosis.[2] For example, farmers have a high risk of osteoarthrosis of the hips, cotton pickers experience degenerative changes of the fingers, miners have elbow and knee problems, and some foundry occupations where heavy, vibrating tools are used are connected with arthrosis of the elbow. The cause does not seem to be hard labor alone, but a combination of heavy work and repetitive activity.[51]

Indicators of Morbidity and Their Measurement

As already mentioned, low-back pain is a variety of different disorders rather than a single entity.[35] A prolapsed lumbar disc may have quite another etiology than, for example, spondylosis, muscle spasms, or inflammatory processes. The diagnostic procedures used to differentiate each syndrome are inaccurate even in clinical examinations of single patients, not to speak of epidemiologic series comprising hundreds or thousands of subjects. For example, Kersley[23] found it impossible to classify more than 60% of a series of 404 patients with chronic back pain, even in a thorough examination. Epidemiologic surveys can rarely, if ever, afford such examination. Follow-up studies, in particular, would require simple and reliable tests, not only for discriminating between the various syndromes causing low-back pain, but also for providing repeatable assessment of the condition of the back. Such tests do not exist. Ethical considerations often prevent the use of certain examinations (e.g., radiographic ones) for clinically symptomless subjects. In case-referent studies, where the number of patients is far smaller, more elaborate examinations can be used, and ethical restrictions are fewer because "cases" are ill. Nevertheless, large cohort studies can hardly afford to devote more than 10 to 15 min to each subject, and all tests must be completely safe. A serious problem is also the lack of good methods for measuring a condition quantitatively.

Example 5. A specially trained physiotherapist carried out a detailed clinical examination of the backs of 298 active concrete reinforcement workers in Uusimaa Province in southern Finland in 1972. Five years later, 252 active concrete reinforcement workers from the same region were examined. The second time the examinations were carried out by two other physiotherapists who were trained by the physiotherapist from the first phase of the study. Every effort was made to make the examinations in the two phases identical. Written instructions including classification criteria for the findings were given to the new examiners by the old examiner, and the first examiner practiced the examination routines with the two new ones on a sample of volunteers. Standardized forms were used to record the findings. Considerable discrepancies were obtained in the prevalences of various clinical findings between the two phases of the study. The prevalence of thoracic scoliosis was 38 vs 65% (1972 vs 1977), enhanced lumbar lordosis 23 vs 14%, pelvic tilting 39 vs 29%, irregular motion in forward bending 38 vs 18%, spasticity of the back muscles 41 vs 22%, decreased abdominal muscle strength 43 vs 5%, and decreased back muscle strength 27 vs 3%. The two samples were similar in age and work experience. Thus the discrepancies indicated poor reliability and repeatability of the clinical examination methods used.[50]

Unfortunately, the history of back-related painful disorders is also unreliable because subjects tend to forget their symptoms and related events, even major ones such as hospitalization.

Example 6. In a prospective questionnaire study of low back trouble, 2222 men representing machine operators, carpenters, and office workers responded to a baseline postal questionnaire (Riihimäki, unpublished results).[55] Three years later an identical questionnaire was mailed to all the respondents. The "forgetting rate"' was defined as the proportion of men who in the follow-up phase answered "no" to a question of ever having had low-back trouble out of those who had answered "yes" to the same question in the first examination. The forgetting rate was 26% for sciatic pain (low-back pain radiating to the legs), 40% for lumbago (sudden attack of low-back pain), 35% for other low-back trouble, and 34% for hospitalization due to a back disease. The forgetting rate, for example, for sciatic pain was related to age and occupation; the forgetting rate was 49% for 25- to 29 year-olds, 19% for 35- to 39-year-olds, and 24% for 45- to 49-year-olds. It was 22% for machine operators, 28% for carpenters, and 31% for office workers.

Such occupation- and age-dependent differences in the variation of the forgetting rates easily leads to bias when the relative risk of sciatic pain is estimated for different occupational groups.

There are also considerable constitutional differences between subjects, including: (1) macroanatomical features such as the size of the spinal canal, bony anomalies, and legs of different lengths; (2) differences between the various collagens—there are about 120 types of collagen—and the composition of the glucoseaminoglycans; (3) natural motor skill, which varies between subjects; (4) variation in muscular strength (the effects of this variation may be either beneficial or harmful because very strong muscles may expose the spine to excessive strain); and (5) variations in psychological properties such as risk-taking and neuroticism. These factors, alone or together, often result in variations whose effects can be much greater than that of the occupational factors under study.

The study of neck and upper-limb disorders, especially disorders that require a long exposure time or repeated small traumas to develop, also encounters several problems. Acute conditions such as peritendinitis and the tennis elbow syndrome can more easily be related to current occupational activities.

In the face of these difficulties, epidemiologic surveys are difficult to plan and must compromise between validity and feasibility. The development of standardized interviews and questionnaires for symptoms is an urgent task. However, the diagnosis cannot rely only on symptoms. Objective examinations should also be standardized (how to assess pain and tenderness, how to ensure repeatability of measurements of mobility, etc.). For example, although seemingly consistent and detailed criteria have been proposed for epicondylitis, achieving repeatability of the examinations has proved difficult. Problems arise because neither the questions on symptoms nor the methods for performing single tests (e.g., location and force of palpation, positioning of the arm in functional tests) have been sufficiently standardized, in spite of some attempts.[49]

Example 7. A study of slaughterhouse workers was so designed that a trained physiotherapist first gave each subject a preplanned physical examination and interviewed the subjects on the same occasion.[48] The screening diagnosis was made according to a predetermined set of criteria. According to these criteria, for example, the epicondylitis syndrome was defined as "local pain during rest and/or movement, local tenderness at the lateral/medial epicondyle, pain during resisted extension/flexion of the wrist and fingers.'' If the screening diagnosis was positive, the subject was remitted for additional tests, which were made by a physician. In the case of elbow pain, these tests comprised measurement of the free and painless range of movement, palpation of the olecranon bursa, palpation of the radial nerve at the edge of the superficial supinator muscle (the arcade of Frohse), and measurement of the strength of middle-finger extension. The criteria for a clinical diagnosis were also preset. In the case of epicondylitis, they were the same as for the screening diagnosis, but for some other disorders they were more elaborated. The thorough physical examination did not reveal many cases of disorders not found by the epidemiologic screening method, with the exception of carpal ganglia.

In the study in the preceding example, it was concluded that the validity of the screening methods used could not be tested, as the clinical and screening diagnoses were based partly on the same tests. Objective findings occurred only rarely in the absence of subjective symptoms. Hence only an interview of the subject's symptoms could constitute the screening procedure, and would therefore reduce efforts and costs in field surveys. However, in elderly persons, degenerative changes cause symptoms and signs that cannot be singled out in a physical examination. Thus the method is best suited for young populations.

The diagnosis of osteoarthrosis is also difficult in epidemiologic studies, not the least because radiographic examinations, which would be necessary, may currently be considered unethical in the case of ''healthy'' individuals. If radiographic examinations cannot be used in an epidemiologic study, the diagnosis must rely on a history of pain and the occurrence of tenderness and mobility restriction, all nonspecific and inaccurate measurements. Furthermore, in osteoarthrosis mobility measurements and radiographic examinations are often conflicting. An alternative approach would be a dynamic, population-based case-referent study in which the work histories of patients with diagnosed osteoarthrosis of some specific joint(s) are compared with those of subjects without the disease. Such an approach would give relative risks for different worker populations and thus identify dangerous tasks. However, avoiding recall bias in such a setting would be difficult indeed.

Assessment of Exposure

Assessing a lifetime history of ''exposure'' is a difficult problem in studies of back pain. In real life, the exposure of the back to various types of trauma, strain, and stress is usually long and diversified. Standardized exposure ratings have not been developed, and even if they existed, the recall of the subjects would probably not be accurate enough to account for a lifetime history of exposure. While some exposures, such as trauma, may cause immediate effects (trauma, of course, can also initiate later effects), others, such as whole-body vibration, may cause symptoms after a long induction period.

Other exposures, such as lifting, may or may not have latent periods before chronic low-back pain results. Often there are combinations of different exposures, and, to complicate matters even more, occupational exposures are frequently confounded by leisure-time exposure such as sports injuries and strain during holiday gardening. In addition, both work and, especially, leisure-time activities, if physiological, can have beneficial effects. This complicated pattern indeed makes the assessment of the occupational etiologic fraction a hard task.

Similar problems are encountered in the study of disorders of the neck and upper limbs and also of arthrosis, especially for disorders which require a long exposure time or repeated small traumas to develop. More acute disorders, such as peritendinitis and the tennis elbow syndrome, can more easily be related to current occupational activities. Thorough and detailed job descriptions are a great help in studies of such disorders. Several methods have been used for exposure assessment, none of them completely satisfactory.[14] They include:

- Static biomechanical models
- Dynamic biomechanical models
- Measurements of energy consumption
- Questionnaires
- Ergonomic assessments
- Registration of work load
- The ARBAN multimoment method
- Ovako Working Posture Analyzing System (OWAS)
- Posture targeting
- Poor working posture (PWP)
- Arbeitswissenschaftliche Erhebungsverfahren zur Tätigkeitsanalyse (AET)

The problems with these methods are that they measure present, not past, exposure and that many of them are time-consuming.

Although many methods for systematically describing manual work have been developed, the analysis of work methods is difficult and laborious. Work movements are many and complex even for monotonous manual tasks. Therefore the study of such exposure is time-consuming and difficult to standardize and relate to measures of disease.

Other Validity Aspects

The study of musculoskeletal disorders, especially of low-back pain, poses several other validity problems. Because these disorders are painful, they cause highly selective turnover out of work with demands on the musculoskeletal system. Such selection invalidates most or all cross-sectional studies, especially since less demanding tasks, often used for contrast, by no means exert such selective power. Hence, in a cross-sectional study, mere selection (and lack of it or selection with an opposite direction in the reference group) can partly or totally mask work-related low-back pain and other musculo-skeletal disorders. It is true that many researchers have nevertheless shown an exceptionally high frequency of, for example, low-back pain in heavy work, but such findings must reflect endurable disorders, not the more severe manifestations, and especially not those leading to incapacity.

Selection is a problem also in longitudinal studies because those with the most severe manifestations tend to quit too early to become classified as having "heavy" or "long-term" exposure. From a practical viewpoint a high turnover also creates difficulties in tracing all members of the study population. However, prospective cohort studies can, if well-designed, be both valid and informative for the study of disorders with short latency, such as traumas, tenosynovitis, and the tennis elbow syndrome. Finally, causation and aggravation are often difficult, if at all possible, to differentiate between—a problem which hampers etiologic research, in particular.

Altogether it may be a mistake to treat low-back pain as a research topic, as though it were an illness. It is, in fact, a complaint with a great number of different causes, not an illness. Therefore research validity would improve if a definitive diagnosis of the anomaly of interest could be arrived at.[33] This requirement would presuppose quite another approach to the epidemiology of low-back pain and would demand much more clinical input and also time-consuming diagnostic procedures. A case-referent design could then, for practical reasons, become the only workable option. These critical remarks should, however, not hinder the planning and implementation of sound studies; the preceding discussion is intended to indicate how difficult the problem can be and how many aspects one must take care of. It attempts, furthermore, to warn the reader against drawing conclusions that are too far-reaching from less well-executed studies. It should also, perhaps, discourage the initiation of studies which, from the very beginning, are doomed to failure.

CORONARY HEART DISEASE

Work-Related Risk Factors

Coronary heart disease (CHD) is the major contributor to cardiovascular and even overall mortality in most industrialized countries. Some well-known major risk factors explain about half of its occurrence. These include age, gender, serum cholesterol value, blood pressure, and tobacco smoking. The other half of the risk includes less well-established factors such as life-style variables, physical inactivity, personality type, diabetes, and social support.[21] Even so, the entire etiology has not been explained, and work-related factors may well play an important role. Several are already known, and others certainly await their identification.

The various *chemical exposures* that have been linked to cardiovascular morbidity have recently been reviewed.[26] These include carbon disulfide, which is atherogenic and, in addition, causes sudden death; organic nitrates, which cause both CHD and sudden death at withdrawal from exposure; arsenic, which has been shown to cause a dose-dependent increase in cardiovascular mortality; and organic solvents, which may cause arrythmias. Carbon monoxide at least aggravates angina pectoris; its role in the causation of CHD is probably insignificant. Cadmium and lead have been accused of causing hypertension; the data are inconclusive, however. Both heat stress and exposure to cold have been linked to cardiovascular morbidity.[27]

Extremes of *heat and humidity* can have strong effects on the cardiovascular system, especially in subjects with underlying organic disease. Acclimatization to hot environments usually takes place within 10 days among healthy subjects, but persons with impaired myocardial function may not be able to respond to heat exposure by increasing cardiac output. In spite of the outspoken effects of heat on cardiovascular performance, especially in persons with cardiovascular disease, there is little if any epidemiologic evidence suggesting increased cardiovascular mortality in populations exposed to high temperatures at work. It is possible that persons with cardiovascular disease are at increased risk for complications, but causative effects of heat have not been shown.

Exposure to *cold* also causes cardiovascular responses. These include anoxia and vasoconstriction, which result in an increased work load. Many patients with coronary heart disease are sensitive to cold. They respond with an elevation of the heart rate and blood pressure. The threshold for angina attacks is lowered. It has been repeatedly shown that cold weather increases coronary mortality. For example, in northern Finland the mortality from coronary infarction depended both on the month and the average temperature.[36] Mortality was more than 20% higher in December, January, and February than in July and August. The effect was especially marked for those over 50 years of age. Controlled cohort studies on workers occupationally exposed to cold are lacking, however.

Physical Activity and Work Stress

Cardiovascular morbidity in relation to physical activity has recently been reviewed.[21,27] Physical activity has a proved beneficial effect on several biochemical and circulatory parameters involved in the pathogenesis of CHD. Many studies have also indicated that physical activity protects against the disease itself.[21,27] About two-thirds of the published studies show a positive relationship between physical inactivity and CHD risk. The better the quality of the study, the clearer the relationship. The median relative risk for CHD is 1.9 for inactive persons when all studies are taken into consideration and 2.4 if only the best studies are included.[27] However, other life-style factors associated with physical activity may explain part of the difference.[21] Furthermore, the risk of dying of CHD is strongly elevated during and soon after strenuous exercise.

Well-controlled studies have shown an increased risk for CHD among certain types of shift workers as compared with day workers. Other studies have not been able to demonstrate such an effect of shift work.[27] Much of the confusion is probably due to selection bias and other uncontrolled errors in design in the poorer studies.[1] Such errors tend to mask a true effect. The negative studies have not properly considered the whole population, or have they differentiated the morbidity with respect to the amount of exposure.[1,27] The better the study design, the higher the relative risk. One of the best studies published showed an overall rate ratio of 1.4 with a clear gradient for length of exposure.[25] This result is consistent with those of other studies of high quality.[27] The effect of shift work on CHD could be directly mediated through the neuroendocrine system, or it could be indirectly due to adverse smoking and eating habits, induced by an irregular life-style. Well-designed, prospective studies are still needed to provide a more convincing answer to this question.

The literature on the role of work stress in the pathogenesis of CHD is conflicting. Work stress is often coupled to stress in one's private life. Moreover, different individuals experience stress in different ways, and therefore objective measurements of "exposure" to stress are difficult. The classical work by Karasek[20] was a major step forward in the clarification of concepts. According to him "stressors" refer to conditions in the environment that can cause stress. Their common characteristics are (1) lack of control, (2) lack of meaning, (3) lack of predictability, (4) over- and understimulation, and (5) conflict. Stress can either influence the cardiovascular system directly through psychophysiological processes or indirectly by inducing stress-related behavior such as excessive smoking and eating. In general, the studies testing Karasek's model have found a relationship between stress and cardiovascular disease. The relative risk for this disease group varied in the different studies from 1.3 to about 4, the highest rate ratios reported in the best studies.[27] Other types of studies have also shown a connection between stress and an increased incidence of cardiovascular disease. Examples of conditions imposing increased risk are insecurity, frustration, competition, irregular work hours, strenuous repetitive physical effort, and time-limit urgency.[27]

Indicators of Morbidity and Their Measurement

CHD has probably been studied epidemiologically more than any other disease. Hence cardiovascular epidemiology has served as a model for the epidemiologic study of chronic diseases in general. However, most of the work done concerns the natural history and general risk factors of CHD, and the impact of occupational factors has not always been sufficiently considered.

The work-relatedness of cardiovascular diseases can be studied epidemiologically at the following three levels:

1. Mortality
2. Morbidity (with infarctions, strokes, disability, electrocardiographic changes at rest and after exercise, angina, and hypertension as the end point)
3. Risk factors (blood lipids, diabetes, obesity, hypertension as a precursor of stroke and CHD, physical inactivity, etc.)

In studies on the connection between work-related risk factors and cardiovascular morbidity, risk factors that are extrinsic to the possible work-relatedness, such as age or smoking, must also be measured and controlled as potential confounders.

Occupational cardiovascular mortality can be studied through the use of national registers in countries with satisfactory death registration. The crudest method is to compare mortality for broad occupational categories. This procedure is followed routinely in the United Kingdom; the occupational mortality statistics published by the Registrar General have been well known for more than 100 years. Currently, such statistics are reviewed in relation to occupational information from the preceding decennial censuses.[12] A study from Finland has shown rather wide variations (SMR 67--131) for cardiovascular mortality between broad occupational categories.[42] However, since social and life-style factors are interwoven with occupational factors and since the registered occupational categories are very broad, such studies are not very conclusive. At most they can suggest connections. However, more probably they mask existing differences between narrower subcategories of workers because of their crudeness.

Ad hoc cohort studies are therefore needed to acquire more accurate data. First, an occupational cohort with a specified exposure, such as, for example, carbon disulfide, shift work, foundry work, a certain level of physical activity (or inactivity), should be defined. The mortality of that cohort can then be checked from national mortality registers and compared with national data, or preferably with those derived from a well-selected reference cohort. If the cohort study is prospective, the researcher can study other indicators of morbidity at the same time, such as nonfatal infarctions, electrocardiographic findings, or angina.

Example 8. In the Finnish study on the effects of carbon disulfide exposure on CHD morbidity, the relative risk during the first 5 years of follow-up was 4.8 for fatal infarctions, 3.7 for all infarctions, and 2.8 for nonfatal infarctions. At the end of the period the prevalence of angina was 2.2 and that for "coronary" ECG's 1.4 times higher than in a reference group of workers from a nearby paper and pulp mill. The use of indicators of different severity of the disease added information to that provided by mere mortality data. It could, for example, be shown that carbon disulfide not only increased the incidence of CHD but also worsened its prognosis.

Prospective studies (e.g., on the effects of shift work upon cardiovascular morbidity) could use a similar approach. Mortality registers become especially important sources of information when the cohort is large, the follow-up is long, and the turnover is great, because tracing all the deceased is difficult or impossible by any other means. In countries having other morbidity registers, "heavy" morbidity such as infarctions and reasons for disability pensions can be studied in a similar way.

Of the milder indicators of CHD, angina and electrocardiographic changes have been studied the most. The questionnaire on angina, developed by WHO, has gained wide use.[54] Likewise, hardly any morbidity study would consider leaving out electrocardiography, either at rest of after standardized exercise. Blind coding of electrocardiographic changes, especially those indicating past infarction or ischemia, according to the so-called Minnesota code and its later revisions,[5] has been recommended during the last two decades. Although individual diagnoses cannot be made on the basis of isolated electrocardiographic findings only, this method—which employs technicians as coders—takes care of observer bias and ensures an objective reading by eliminating more or less well-founded "clinical impressions." More recently, computerized techniques for the coding of electrocardiograms have been developed and introduced; this step has further improved the quality of readings.

Blood pressure measurements are often included in surveys of cardiovascular morbidity. Although the measurement itself is simple, there are methodologic requirements that should be attended to. The manometer should be well calibrated and the cuff broad and long. The position of the subject should always be the same (either sitting or supine) and a rest of 15 to 20 min should precede the measurement. The reading of the diastolic pressure should be standardized (e.g., disappearance of Korotkoff's sound). Blood pressure fluctuates normally during the day, and the examination itself may cause it to rise. Repeated measurements may therefore be needed.

The selection of morbidity parameters in cardiovascular surveys is not guided only by scientific considerations. The vast amount of cardiologic examination methods available may tempt the investigator to use several tests, preferably modern and sophisticated ones, on the one hand, while restrictions on funds and the limited availability of technicians act inhibitingly, on the other. An absolute requirement in epidemiologic surveys is, furthermore, that no risk be imposed on the subject. This requirement is stricter than in the clinical setting, in which the patient benefits from the examinations and in which risk considerations are, therefore, different. The requirement of complete safety further restricts the tests that can be recommended for epidemiologic studies; one may even question if, for example, maximal exercise electrocardiography and cold provocation are justified. When selecting tests for a survey, it is crucial to ponder thoroughly what information can be gained from each of the alternative tests. For example, increasing the sensitivity of electrocardiographic examinations through the use of a maximal exercise test may add to the study in some instances; in others, it may not yield any further information. An exercise test causes much extra work and implies, possibly, a slight risk for some subjects. In the Finnish carbon disulfide study, the inclusion of exercise electrocardiography gave no additional information.[16]

However, this conclusion emerged at hindsight — knowing in advance what exactly each examination will yield is not so simple.

Assessment of Exposure

As far as chemical or physical factors are concerned, assessment of exposure is a matter of well-conducted, conventional occupational hygienic measurements. As usual, the main problem is how to secure retrospective exposure data, because at least the atherogenetic process preceding cardiovascular attacks is a slow, chronic event which should be related to exposure over a long time span.

When the issue is shift work, it is important to describe exactly the specific type of work concerned and not to mix too many different systems under "exposure." Any study of the effect of work-related factors upon cardiovascular morbidity should, of course, measure the known major risk factors for this disease group so that they can be statistically controlled. These measurements cause much extra input in terms of manpower and economic resources, but are nevertheless unavoidable to ensure validity of the study.

As mentioned earlier, occupational factors may be either direct or indirect causes of cardiovascular disease. When planning a study, the researcher should be well aware of which mechanism is operating, because the study design is influenced by it.

Example 9. If the issue is to study whether or not shift work causes CHD, mental stress is a possible etiologic factor. Controlling stress statistically would then block the effect. Therefore, the reference group should be one without exceptional stress.

Example 10. If, on the other hand, the question is whether exposure to carbon disulfide causes CHD, mental stress is an extrinsic factor (probably) not related to the causal chain. In this situation, mental stress should be controlled as a potential confounder. In other words, the reference group should be exposed to the same amount of stress (e.g., in the form of shift work) as the exposed group, or different stress levels should be analyzed separately.

Other Validity Aspects

The great experience gained from coronary epidemiology, in general, should also be utilized in the design of valid studies on work-related problems. The accumulated knowledge of the relative importance of the "heavy" risk factors, namely, smoking, hypertension, and hyperlipemia, as well as of others, such as diabetes, physical inactivity, or gout, helps to identify and control potential confounders in a study on work-related coronary morbidity. The better the control of the nonoccupational factors, the greater the sensitivity of a study to detect work-related factors. However, as mentioned before, matching on intermediates in the etiologic chain leads to the masking of a true effect and should therefore not be done. For example, in the Finnish carbon disulfide study, blood pressure and the serum cholesterol level were measured but not controlled statistically. The reason was earlier suggestions that some of the mechanisms by which carbon disulfide may increase coronary morbidity could be intermediated through hypertension and hyperlipemia.[16]

Selection is another problem. CHD is known to cause a strong healthy worker effect,[32] partly because early symptoms may force the workers to quit or primarily to seek a light job and partly because it is possible to identify high-risk individuals at an early stage. Such persons may not be hired, or they may selectively become unemployed, especially during periods of economic depression. This possibility leads to lower mortality for the remaining workers; milder manifestations, especially angina, also become underrepresented. Therefore it is important to define and use a reference group in which the same types of selective forces operate.

Studies on shift work and coronary and other cardiovascular morbidity are said to be especially vulnerable to selection bias. Rapid turnover of workers may be due to health selection; in addition, the turnover causes short exposure times for most of the cohort and therefore dilutes the results.[1] Selection into shift work may also be difficult to control for. To remedy this problem, worksites with few possibilities for transfer should be favored. Furthermore, the analyses should be made separately for different lengths of employment in shift work, and this requirement increases the demands on cohort size. Big enterprises, located in remote areas, such as some paper mills in the Nordic countries or British Columbia, could provide good opportunities for research, because there are usually few alternative job opportunities in such places. The case-referent design has perhaps not received enough attention in cardiovascular epidemiology. This design is not optimal for all indicators (e.g., sudden death, for which the work history must be obtained from the next-of-kin). However, it could be useful if the cases were, for example, survivors of coronary infarctions. Especially when many etiologic factors at a time should be studied or controlled for, this approach improves the cost efficiency of the study since exposure data need to be gathered only for the cases and their referents, and not for the whole study base. Therefore a more thorough penetration is possible. For example, information on psychosocial factors could be obtained in great detail. However, the serious problem with this approach is how to control recall bias, which may be difficult whenever the interview concerns mental stress. Another problem is that data on some coronary risk factors, such as predisease blood lipids and blood pressure, may not be obtainable and their control as potential confounders would therefore be impossible.

BEHAVIORAL RESPONSES AND PSYCHOSOMATIC SYMPTOMS

Sources of Stress at Work

Several work-related factors can cause mental stress. Important stressors are inadverse ergonomic conditions, shift work, work overload, work underload combined with boredom, underutilization of psychological abilities, discrepancy between expectations and capabilities, on the one hand and the role in the organization, on the other, unsatisfactory career development, physical danger, poor personal relations at work, and bad organizational structure and atmosphere.[9,52] Physical factors such as exposure to noise often act as stressors; some chemical exposures, such as heavy metals and organic solvents, may cause neurotoxic symptoms which can be confused with symptoms of stress.

It is important to realize that work-related stress and psychosocial problems in the domestic sphere are often interwoven, and aggravate each other. Together they may lead to unhealthy behavior and thus both directly and indirectly increase morbidity. A holistic approach must therefore be taken in epidemiologic studies on work-related psychosocial problems. The rapid changes which are now taking place in worklife all over the world (e.g., industrialization, urbanization, migration, automation, and computerization), combined with aging of the work force at least in the industrialized countries, accentuate many psychosocial problems and increase the relative weight of psychosocial factors in occupational health.

Psychosomatic and Behavioral Symptomatology as Consequences of Work-Related Stress

All over the world, psychosomatic and behavioral symptoms are extremely common in the working population.[19,29] For example, in Sweden every third adult suffers from symptoms such as malaise, sleep disorders, fatigue, dejection, or anxiety; every seventh is exhausted at the end of the workday; and half of the men and three-quarters of the women suffer from mental breakdown on one or more occasions before the age of 60. Ten percent of the men have alcohol-related problems and the rate of suicide is 2.03 per 10,000.[29] According to several reports from different countries, about half of the working population is unsatisfied with their jobs and three-fourths of those who consult psychiatrists relate their problems to lack of job satisfaction or inability to relax.[29]

Work-related stress may act on health either directly or by inducing an unhealthy life-style. Smoking has been shown to be associated with tension and anxiety and also with high levels of quantitative work load.[31,52] Alcohol abuse can be also related to work stress and a feeling of insufficiency; it can be a method of escaping stress. Overeating is often related to anxiety, and lack of physical exercise can be related to psychoneurotic exhaustion or to too heavy a work load (e.g., holding two jobs). All these habits are known to influence health in a negative way; for example, the connection between smoking and a number of diseases such as coronary heart disease, several forms of cancer, and gastrointestinal disorders is well known. Alcohol abuse causes many disorders, among them excess overall mortality, cirrhosis of the liver, cardiovascular disorders, damage to the nervous system, accidents, and suicide. Direct psychosomatic effects of work-related stress include mental disorders, mass psychogenic illness, gastrointestinal symptoms (e.g., dyspepsia, indigestion, and heartburn), cardiovascular symptoms (e.g., palpitation, arrythmias and chest pain, as well as hypertension and coronary heart disease), respiratory symptoms (e.g., hyperventilation), central nervous system symptoms (e.g., neurotic reactions, insomnia, weakness, faintness and headache), and genital symptoms (e.g., frigidity and impotence).[29] All these manifestations can be used as indicators of effect in studies on work-related stress.

The pathogenetic mechanisms for these reactions are certainly complicated and manyfold. Two broad categories of mechanisms have been considered particularly relevant, namely, neuroendocrine reactions, involving the hypothalamo–adrenomedullary and hypophyseo–adrenocortical axes, and reactions in the immune system.[29,52] For example, the level of catecholamines in blood or urine has been used for assessing stress. Other biochemical measurements indicating disturbances in these systems could be developed for use as indicators of stress in epidemiologic studies.

Problems in Study Design

Many studies have searched for associations between psychosocial factors at work and health. They have mostly been explorative and cross-sectional in design; causal inferences are difficult to draw from such studies. By contrast, longitudinal etiologic studies with good validity have been rare, and the same can be said of interventions. The small number of such etiologic studies probably has to do with the great input of resources needed; also the complexity of the situation is a problem that makes the design of a valid study extremely difficult and expensive.

Research on behavioral responses and psychosomatic symptomatology generally relies on the use of interviews and questionnaires. These techniques can yield valid results only in the hands of skilled and experienced researchers, but they appear so simple and uncomplicated that there is danger that they will also be used by researchers without the necessary skills. Most situations giving rise to behavioral and psychosomatic symptomatology, be it aggressiveness, depression, insomnia, or psychosomatic diseases, such as hypertension or peptic ulcer, are so full of emotional conflicts that unbiased responses to the questions may be difficult to obtain. Because the general social environment also has a great impact on the entire individual, it is always necessary to incorporate many questions relating to the general life situation into all surveys on occupational risks. This necessity adds to the demands on the qualifications of the investigator; it greatly increases the number of test variables and thereby also renders the questionnaires/interviews laborious to administer and cumbersome to analyze.

The effect variables are often diffuse and nonspecific, and therefore strictly standardized and validated diagnostic criteria are required. Reliable diagnostics can be achieved for "heavy" end points such as coronary infarction, suicide, or peptic ulcer, but milder manifestations such as insomnia, headache, or vertigo can be difficult or impossible to define in a valid and concise way. Furthermore, the causal chain from exposure to effect is not always straightforward. For example, when work stress first causes an overconsumption of tobacco and alcohol, this reaction can be considered an "effect" as such. However, this abuse can also indirectly (from the point of view of stress) cause increased morbidity, as has already been discussed. Such complicated interactions must be understood well before any study is initiated, and allowance for such circumstances must be made both at the planning stage (collection of enough information and sufficient contrasts between subgroups) and at the data analysis stage (sophisticated multivariate statistical methods). Whenever objective methods of assessing the psychological work load are available, for example, the German so-called AET method,[41] they should be used. For example, factors such as the level of the work demands, the number of stimuli, the repetitiveness of the tasks, and the degree of control over the work situation can be assessed objectively. However, subjective assessments of how the subjects perceive themselves in relation to the work situation are usually the main source of information, because many work "exposures," such as social interaction, are not measurable objectively at all.

The choice of a valid reference group is especially difficult in psychosocial epidemiology where many background variables outside the work situation must be controlled. There are many unpredictable social changes in human life that may affect the study group and the referents in different ways, the result being a distortion of an initially sound comparison, especially in a study with a longitudinal design. From a practical viewpoint, it may be impossible to collect all the relevant background data before the groups are formed, so that controlling any intervening and confounding factors then becomes a problem for the data analysis. This type of control is not possible without detailed information on potential confounders.

Selection is particularly difficult to control in psychosocial studies. Most people choose their occupation at least partly on psychological grounds, and factors such as motivation, personality, and initial intellectual or psychomotor capacity play an important role. These are likely to be far more important at job entry than factors related to health. In the same way, selection out of a job often depends on psychological factors, although the importance of medical aspects is likely to be greater than at entry. Finding a reference group in which the initial forces of selection into the job, the relevant job characteristics, and the forces determining selection out of it are all similar can often prove to be an impossible task.

The use of intraindividual comparisons overcomes some of these difficulties, but this approach requires a longitudinal design, with or without an intervention. Furthermore, a before–after evaluation can introduce other biases, and a reference group is therefore usually also required. Prospective longitudinal studies, although also struggling against uncontrollable bias, certainly give more reliable data than cross-sectional ones, but the costs can easily become formidable because repeated measurements of many variables are required. Furthermore, because of a predicted loss of subjects due to dropout, the initial study groups must be much larger than actually needed to measure an effect. Cost therefore often restricts the use of a prospective design.

REFERENCES

1. Åkerstedt, T., A. Knutsson, L. Alfredsson, and T. Theorell. "Shift work and cardiovascular disease," *Scand. J. Work Environ. Health* 10:409-14 (1984).
2. Anderson, J. A. D. "Arthrosis and its relation to work," *Scand. J. Work Environ. Health* 10:429-3 (1984).
3. Association of Schools of Public Health. "Proposed National Strategies for the Prevention of Leading Work-Related Diseases and Injuries," Association of Schools of Public Health (1986).
4. Bigos, S., M. Battié, D. Spengler, L. Fisher, and A. Nachemson. "Back injuries in industry: a retrospective study. III. Employee-related factors," *Spine* 3:252-6 (1986).
5. Blackburn, H., A. Keys, E. Simonson, P. Rautaharju, and S. Punsar. "The electrocardiogram in population studies: a classification system, *Circulation* 21:1160-75 (1960).
6. Brooks, S. M. "Bronchial asthma of occupational origin," *Scand. J. Work Environ Health* 3:53-72 (1977).
7. Brooks, S. M. "Bronchial asthma of occupational origin," in *Environmental and Occupational Medicine,* V. N. Rom, Ed. (Boston, MA: Little, Brown, 1983) pp. 233-50.
9. Cooper, C. L., and M. Davidson. "Sources of stress at work and their relation to stressors in non-working environments," in *Psychosocial Factors at Work and Their Relation to Health,* Kalimo, R., M. A. El-Batawi, and C. L. Cooper, Eds. (Geneva: WHO, 1987) pp. 99-111.
10. Eisen, A. E., D. H. Wegman, and T. A. Louis. "Effects of selection in a prospective study of forced expiratory volume in Vermont granite workers," *Am. Rev. Respir. Dis.* 128:587-91 (1983).
11. El-Batawi, M. A. "Work-related diseases: a new program of the World Health Organization," *Scand. J. Work Environ. Health* 10:341-6 (1984).
12. Fox, A. J., and A. M. Adelstein. "Occupational mortality: work or way of life? *J. Epidemiol. Community Health* 32:73-8 (1978).
13. Hagberg M., and D. H. Wegman. "Prevalence rates and odds ratios of shoulder-neck diseases in different occupational groups," *Br. J. Ind. Med.* 44:602-10 (1987).

14. Hansson, T. *Ländryggsbesvär och arbete*. (Stockholm: Swedish Work Environment Fund, 1989.)

16. Hernberg, S., T. Partanen, C.-H. Nordman, and P. Sumari. "Coronary heart disease among workers exposed carbon disulphide," *Br. J. Ind. Med.* 27:313-325 (1970).

17. IARC. "Monographs on the Evaluation of Carcinogenic Risks to Humans, Suppl 7," Overall evaluations of carcinogenicity: an updating of IARC monographs volumes 1 to 42. (Lyon: IARC, 1987).

18. ILO. "Guidelines for the Use of ILO International Classification of Radiographs of Pneumoconioses." (Geneva:ILO,1980.) (Occupational Safety and Health Ser., No. 22).

19. Kalimo R, M. A. El-Batawi, and C. L. Cooper, Eds. *Psychological Factors at Work and Their Relation to Health* (Geneva: WHO, 1987).

20. Karasek, R. A. "Job demands, job decision latitude, and mental strain: implications for job redesign," *Adm. Sci. Q.* 24:285-308 (1979).

21. Karvonen, M. J. "Physical activity and cardiovascular morbidity," *Scand. J. Work Environ. Health* 10:389-95 (1984).

22. Keimig, D. G., P. R. Pomrehn, and L. F. Burmeister. "Respiratory symptoms and pulmonary function in welders of mild steel: a cross-sectional study," *Am. J. Ind. Med.* 4:489-99 (1983).

23. Kersley, G. D. "Back pain: its problems and treatments," *Curr. Med. Res. Opin.* 6:27-32 (1979).

24. Keskinen, H., O. Tupasela, U. Tiikkainen, C.-H. Nordman. "Experiences of specific IGE in asthma due to isocyanates," *Clin. Allergy* 18:547-604 (1988).

25. Knutsson, A., T. Åkerstedt, B. G. Johnsson, and K. Orth-Gomer, "Increased risk of ischaemic heart disease in shift workers," *Lancet* 2:89-92 (1986).

26. Kristensen, T. J. "Cardiovascular diseases and the work environment. A critical review of the epidemiologic literature on chemical factors. *Scand. J. Work Environ. Health* 15:245-64 (1989).

27. Kristensen, T. J. "Cardiovascular disease and the work environment. A critical review of the epidemiologic literature on nonchemical factors. *Scand. J. Work Environ. Health* 15:165-79 (1989b).

28. Kurppa, K., P. Waris, and P. Rokkanen. "Tennis elbow: lateral elbow pain syndrome," *Scand. J. Work Environ. Health* 6 (Suppl. 3):15-8 (1979).

29. Levi, L. "Psychosomatic disease as a consequence of occupational stress," in *Psychosocial Factors at Work and Their Relation to Health,* Kalimo, R., M. A. El-Batawi, and C. L. Cooper, Eds. (Geneva: WHO 1987), pp. 78-91.

30. Malker, H. S. R., J. K. McLaughlin, B. K. Malker, B. J. Stone, J. A. Weiner, J. L. E. Erickson, and W. J. Blot. "Occupational risk for pleural mesothelioma in Sweden, 1961-79," *J. Natl. Cancer Inst.* 74:61 (1985).

31. McCrae, R. R., P. T. Costa, and R. Bossé. "Anxiety, extroversion and smoking, *Br. J. Soc. Clin. Psychol.* 17:269-73 (1978).

32. McMichael, A. J. "Standardized mortality ratios and the 'healthy worker effect': Scratching beneath the surface," *J. Occup. Med.* 18:165 (1976).

33. Miettinen, O. S., and J. J. Caro. "Medical research on a complaint: orientation and priorities, *Ann. Intern. Med.* 21:399-401 (1989).

34. Murphy, R. L. H., Jr. "Industrial disease with asthma," in *Bronchial Asthma: Mechanisms·and Therapeutics,* Weiss, E. B., and M. S. Segal, Eds. (Boston, MA: Little, Brown, 1976) pp. 517-536.

35. Nachemson, A. "A critical look at conservative treatment for low back pain," *Eular Bull.* 11(4):234-38 (1982).

36. Näyhä, S. "Short and medium-term variations in mortality in Finland, *Scand. J. Soc. Med.* Suppl. 21 (1981).

37. NIOSH. "Criteria for a Recommended Standard... Occupational Exposure to Diisocyanates." Washington, DC: US Governmental Printing Office, 1978. [DHEW (NIOSH) Publ. No. 78-215.]

38. Nordman, C.-H. "Atopy and work," *Scand. J. Work Environ. Health* 10:481-5 (1984).

39. Pepys, J., and B. J. Hatchcroft. "Bronchial provokation tests in etiological diagnosis of asthma," *Am. Rev. Respir. Dis.* 112:829-36 (1975).

40. Pukkala, E., L. Teppo, and T. Hakulinen. "Keuhkosyöpäsairastavuus eri ammattialoilla Suomessa," *Sos lääket aikak* 1:363 (1979).

41. Rohmert, W., and K. Landau. "Das Arbeitswissenschaftliche Erhebungsverfahren zur Tätigkeitsanalyse (AET)," *Handbuch und Merkmalheft* (Bern: Huber, 1979.)

42. Sauli, H. "Occupational Mortality in 1971-75," Helsinki: Central Statistical Office of Finland, 1979.

43. Sjögren, B., and U. Ulfvarson. "Respiratory symptoms and pulmonary function among welders working with aluminium, stainless steel and railroad trucks," *Scand. J. Work Environ. Health* 11:27-32 (1985).

44. Sweetnam, P. M., S. W. Taylor, and P. C. Elwood. "Exposure to carbon disulphide and ischaemic heart disease in a viscose rayon factory," *Br. J. Ind. Med.* 44:220-7 (1987).

45. Tolonen, M., S. Hernberg, C.-H. Nordman, S. Goto, K. Sugimoto, and T. Baba. "Angina pectoris, electrocardiographic findings and blood pressure in Finnish and Japanese workers exposed to carbon disulfide, "*Int. Arch. Occup. Environ. Health* 37:249-64 (1976).

46. Troup, J. D. G. "Causes, prediction and prevention of back pain at work," *Scand. J. Work Environ. Health* 10:419-28 (1984).

47. Vainio, H. "Occupational cancer prevention," *J. Cancer Res. Clin. Oncol.* 113:403-412 (1987).

48. Viikari-Juntura, E. "Neck and upper limb disorders among slaughterhouse workers: an epidemiologic and clinical study," *Scand. J. Work Environ. Health* 9:283-90 (1983).

49. Viikari-Juntura, E. "Tenosynovitis, peritendinitis and the tennis elbow syndrome," *Scand. J. Work Environ. Health* 10:443-9 (1984).

50. Wickström, G., J. Nummi, M. Wiikeri, and H. Riihimäki. Betoniraudoittajat. Osa 2. Kliininen tutkimus. Helsinki:1975. Työterveyslaitos, Työterveyslaitoksen tutkimuksia 98. (Engl. summary.)

51. Williams, H. J., and J. R. Ward. "Musculoskeletal occupational syndrome," in *Environmental and Occupational Medicine*, W. N. Rom, Ed. (Boston, MA: Little, Brown, 1983) pp. 351-7.

52. WHO Expert Committee. "Identification and Control of Work-Related Diseases: Report of a WHO Expert Committee," WHO, Geneva, 1985. (WHO Tech. Rept. Ser. No. 714).

53. WHO. "Sixth Report on the World Health Situation," WHO, Geneva, 1980, p. 111.

54. WHO. "Cardiovascular survey methods." 2nd ed., WHO, Geneva, 1982.

55. Riihimäki, H. unpublished results.

CHAPTER 7

Planning a Study: The Study Protocol

WHY IS A STUDY PROTOCOL NEEDED?

An epidemiologic study is usually a large and complex undertaking of long duration, requiring the input of human, organizational, and material resources. Such an endeavor cannot succeed without careful and detailed planning. The study plans of large projects cannot be stored in the minds of the researchers; they must be systematically laid down in the form of a *study protocol*.

The study protocol comprises not only an explicit account of the study plan, but also a detailed diary of the execution of the plan, i.e., how the project is progressing. It should be self-evident that a thorough and detailed protocol is essential for a project that may cost hundreds of thousands, even millions of dollars, but surprisingly many researchers perceive the study protocol as an unnecessary, bureaucratic burden.

Miettinen[2] has stressed five main purposes of the study protocol:

1. Crystallize the project to the researchers themselves. Forcing oneself to write down ideas usually improves them. The procedure requires clarity of thought; messy thinking will not go unnoticed.
2. Give referees the possibility to review the project. This is particularly pertinent whenever the researcher applies for outside funding, and whenever initiation of the project requires formal permission by one's institution.
3. Inform and educate all those taking part in the project, such as technicians and consultants.
4. Ensure that the main researchers do not forget any details of the plan in the course of the study, and secure the continuity of the project in case some key member of the team moves to other tasks or even dies.
5. Document the procedures of the project for the future.

STUDY PLAN

The study plan is a detailed account of what the researchers intend to do. It is an important document, because the fate of the project may stand or fall with it. (Will it be funded? What will the research committee's or the director's decision be?) It is therefore worthwhile to put sufficient time into the planning, to consult senior experts, statisticians, and other specialists, and to discuss all the details with the team members. The results of these efforts should then be carefully recorded and rediscussed, and perhaps revised once again. The written plan must be so complete and detailed that another competent researcher would be able to carry out the project on the basis of the plan.

The study plan should contain the following elements:

0. Summary
1. Background
2. Objectives
3. Study design
4. Methods and procedures
5. Control of confounding
6. Preparation of data and computerization
7. Statistical methods
8. Ethical considerations
9. Publication and information
10. Time schedule
11. Project organization
12. Budget

The *background of the project* is the first item. It summarizes what is already known of the problem, what is not known, and whether there are conflicting views. By this stage the researchers must be well acquainted with the literature on the subject matter and also master the methodology. "Methodology" implies much more than data processing and statistical analysis; it may encompass anything from lung function tests or nerve conduction velocity measurements to the analysis of DNA-adducts. It would be frustrating to realize, when the project is well under way, that the problem had already been solved earlier, or that the methodology was outdated. A study plan in which the first step is labeled "literature survey" reveals that the researchers are ignorant of the subject matter. It is imperative that they know the literature already before they start planning the project. Finally, if the project has a practical, problem-solving purpose, it is recommendable to conclude the background section with an assessment of the social relevance of the study; and of the preventive measures it can lead to.

The *objectives* of the study should then be defined. It is prudent not to list too many objectives, because this may blur one's own thinking and hamper the readers' understanding. No more than three or four primary objectives should be defined. If necessary, these can be further divided into subtitles or secondary objectives.

The study objectives should be well defined, there should be only a few of them, and they should be concise.

The objectives should be unequivocally and intelligibly defined, so that other people can understand exactly what the researchers try to say. When formulating the objectives, it is important for the researchers to realize whether the problem is descriptive (e.g., what is the prevalence of back pain among bus drivers), or whether it is etiological. If it is etiological, the researcher must decide if the objective is qualitative (e.g., does ethylene oxide cause leukemia), or quantitative (e.g., how high is the risk of lung cancer for never-smokers who have been exposed to amosite asbestos at concentrations five times the hygienic standard for more than 20 years). The last-mentioned example, besides being quantitative, also restricts the problem to encompass a single category only (nonsmoking men). If funding and supply of material permit, other subcategories of objectives could also be formulated, such as the risk for smokers, for women (probably it would not be possible to find enough subjects in this category), for lower exposure levels, for shorter exposure times, and so forth. Strict definition of such goals is not only an intellectual exercise, but crucial for determining the size of the study material required and for planning the research strategy. For instance, detailed exposure data must be available, for a quantitative study whereas a qualitative study can do with cruder data, such as classification into exposed and unexposed persons. A purely descriptive study may sometimes require no exposure data at all.

The distinction between a qualitative and a quantitative study is important.

Under *"study material"* one should first define the *study base* and then the *study type*. The study base could, for example, be defined as "20-year follow-up of all men who have been employed for at least 3 years in the period 1951 to 1975 in Dutch steel foundries," or "20 year follow-up of heavily exposed workers in a rock wool plant during a certain time period ('heavily' must be defined)." Next, one has to decide whether everybody belonging to the study base will be included (census), that is, the design will be of a cohort type, or if only cases of the illness of interest and a sample of noncases will be studied, that is, the design will be of a case-referent type. A case-referent design can be utilized from a cohort base or the study base can be the follow-up of a dynamic population during a certain period of time, for example, a whole country during 3 years. The cases can then be defined, for example, as "all cases of primary liver cancer (or female cases only) diagnosed in the whole country and reported to the cancer registry during 1988 to 1990." There can be further refinement of the case definition, such as mention of the case being alive (or dead), having undergone autopsy, having hepatocellular carcinoma only, not being over 75 years of age at death, and so forth. The base population can also be restricted to a smaller geographical region, such as the municipality of Lille, the isle of Guernsey, or the catchment area of the Linköping University Hospital. The referents must belong to the same study base, or otherwise be comparable to the study group, they must be equally well defined, and must be comparable to the cases (see Chapter 5).

The study base should be explicitly defined.

At this stage it is difficult to escape the tricky question of the required study size. Quite often this is determined by the availability of subjects; if the supply is ample, the place for formal power calculations is here (see Chapter 5). A qualitative study requires less material than a quantitative one. The need for subgrouping, based either on exposure classes or confounder classes, is important when considering the size of the material.

A qualitative study requires less material than a quantitative one.

The frequency of the phenomenon of interest in the study base is equally important when judging the required study size. If various methods of prior assessment, either formal or intuitive, or both, suggest that the study, as originally envisaged, will be too small to be informative, everything is not yet lost. One can, for example, lower the level of ambition (in a quantitative study). A two-point design, focusing on the extremes and dismissing intermediate exposure categories, is cost-efficient and should be considered, especially when funds are limited. One can also set up a system with an extended follow-up time, or one can try to organize a multicenter, either national or international, joint program (not recommended to junior researchers; seniors may succeed in this difficult task if they are patient and good diplomats). When everything fails, abandoning the project may be the only option left (however much it hurts).

Multicenter studies are difficult, and can be recommended only if one center cannot carry out the study alone, e.g., because of insufficient material or expertise.

The *collection of material* must be described in great detail. What companies, what type of work, what time periods, what sources of information will be used, will there be problems with regulations on confidentiality? Are the companies willing to participate? What about the unions? The reference material should be described in similar detail. What are the criteria for inclusion into or exclusion from the groups? For example, in a study on neurotoxicity, will diabetics be excluded and, if so, how will diabetes be defined and diagnosed? What about skull trauma in a study on the effects of solvents on the central nervous system?

The admissibility criteria must be defined in cohort studies in terms of minimum exposure, calendar time of exposure, whether or not other exposures are permitted, and so forth. If a case-referent design is adopted, the admissibility criteria for both cases and referents must be well defined. For example, what histological types of cancer will be included, how will the diagnosis be confirmed, what are the criteria for "chronic bronchitis," "neuropathy," "asthma," "prolapse of a lumbar disc," and so forth? What is the reference diagnosis? Are the referents indeed representative of the study base? There are many more questions. Will the study be a field study, a hospital-based study, or a register linkage study? Who will collect the data, for example, from what registers, plants, hospitals, and who will perform the clinical measurements? How will the person-years be counted? How will expected values be computed? What are the reasons for using the general population as the reference (in spite of what was said in Chapter 5 of this book and elsewhere in the modern literature)?

A study plan must be so detailed that an independent researcher could carry out the study based on the plan.

These questions are only examples of how detailed the description of the data acquisition must be. Each project has its own list of questions, so the illustration of all problems that may arise is not possible here. The rule of thumb should be, again, that enough details should be given to make it possible for an outsider to carry out the study on the basis of the study plan. Needless to say, a thorough and detailed description will also impress the reviewers of the funding agency.

The *measuring methods and procedures* should be described in detail. First, one should define what the study deals with at a conceptual level (e.g., exposures, diseases, symptoms, syndromes), then one should describe the methods that will be used to measure the indicators of these entities. Will the indicators describe the entities well enough? For instance, is today's blood lead level a good measure of long-term exposure? Is a specially designed symptom questionnaire specific and sensitive enough to measure, e.g., the neurotoxic effects of solvents? The most central issues of the measuring methods, for example, questionnaires, should be summarized in the plan itself, and the detailed method can be added as an appendix. The methods of quality control should be described. Has the institution taken part in some external program, e.g., in blood lead analyses, and what have the results been?

If there are several observers, e.g., interviewers, there should be an account of how they will be trained and how the inter- and intraobserver error will be measured. Will there be blinding? Routine laboratory methods need not be described in detail, however, but references should be given to the methods used. If X-ray films are part of the study, there should be a description of how they will be read, and of the criteria for "positive" findings. Will there be a panel? How will disagreements be solved? Will sequential films be read without showing their order? Whenever examinations require standardization (e.g., room temperature, fasting, rest in the supine position), this must be mentioned. If a pilot study has already been done, the experiences from it should be summarized if they have bearing on the methods selected or on how the measurements will be performed. Again, details are crucial.

The *control of confounding* should be discussed next. Potential confounders must always be measured, because otherwise their control is not possible. The identification of potential confounders requires good insight into the subject matter. One should remember that chance confounding can occur even in (small) randomized materials.

One should also describe how the information will be *classified and reduced*, how missing information will be treated (e.g., nonrespondents), and what the criteria are for omitting data, for example, illogical or clearly wrong measurements. Omitting data is dangerous, and should in general be avoided, but sometimes it becomes evident that something has gone wrong. For example, it may become evident that a few subjects have given a false history, a series of assays may be wrong because of technical failure, and so on. One has the right to omit such results, but only according to preset criteria. This is not the same as succumbing to the temptation to "modify" the results so that they fit better with the researchers' prior hypothesis.

Classification of the data usually means the grouping of a continuous variable into classes, such as, high, medium, and low, in which case tentative criteria and cut-off points should be given. Classification can also imply definition of the dichotomy between "normal" and "pathological." This criterion should be set in advance, at least broadly.

Errors may arise during the data processing; their control must be described. If the number of variables is great, it is easy to end up with too many tables, making the article unreadable. The data reduction and the formation of summary variables should be outlined. Only the most central findings can be shown in table form—otherwise the author will certainly come up against difficulties in getting the work accepted for publication. By the planning stage one must restrict the amount of data to be collected. Too many details and too many different variables measuring the same conceptual entity result in a waste of time and money without contributing to the yield of the study. It is wise to make sure that computing facilities are available when needed, and that the necessary programs exist. This should be documented. Advance consultation with a computer expert ensures that the forms used will be suitable for automatic data processing.

The *statistical methods* to be used should be mentioned, but details are not necessary for routinely used methods. It is recommended to outline how confounding will be controlled and how errors of measurement will be treated.

A short discussion of *ethical aspects* (see Chapter 8) should be written next. For example, how will the consent of the subjects be obtained and how will they be informed? Are all examinations ethically acceptable? How will confidentiality be guaranteed, and how will the data be stored safely?

An outline of the *publication and information scheme* is needed at the planning stage. Epidemiologic research is of interest not only to epidemiologists and other professionals, but also to decision makers, trade unions, companies, manufacturers, funding agencies, and, sometimes, even to the general public. The information given to the different target groups must be adjusted to fit each one's interests and comprehension capacity. It is worthwhile to plan in advance how the information will be dispersed. Those taking part in a study (the so-called "subjects") have the right to know, especially when medical examinations are involved, not only their personal results but also, at least in general terms, the outcome of the whole study. It is important to time the sequence of information correctly. First, those examined should be informed of their own test results, then summary results (without personal identification) should be given to the companies, the unions, and the funding agency, and only then to the news media. Ideally a peer-reviewed scientific article should have appeared or at least have been accepted for publication before informing the news media. Unfortunately, however, the scientific publishing procedure is so slow that it sometimes may be unethical to withhold urgent results from the public that long. In spite of this, it is important to realize that one's scientific reputation soon becomes questionable if one selects the television as the first forum of "publication."

The right sequence of information to different interest groups should be considered in advance.

A large project usually gives rise to several scientific publications, and it may be useful to outline their contents in advance. At the planning stage it is advisable to agree within the team on who will be responsible, i.e., the first author, of what, and whose names should be listed as coauthors. It is usually not possible to decide the order of names at this stage, because each team member's input to the intellectual process can be judged only after the project has been successfully completed.

The *time schedule* of the project must be worked out thoroughly, in sufficient detail, and realistically. Time scheduling concerns the different operational tasks and resources — human, organizational, and material. It is good practice to outline the tasks and subtasks, and to plan their time flow, as well as the necessary resources required for each. The better all details of the project have been considered, the easier it is to work out the time schedule. Once it has been decided how many subjects will be included, and what methods of examination will be used, the time needed can be estimated rather accurately. At the planning stage one should make sure that statistical and computerizing assistance is available when needed, not merely at some indefinite time in the future. The researcher must also stick to his/her original schedule, to avoid disrupting the consultants' time schemes, which may possibly result in chain reactions affecting other projects. This may mean fighting with one's superiors, or declining attractive invitations to congresses. One should realize that the first data analysis almost always results in further analyses, and these again in new computations. Enough time must be reserved for all of these considerations.

Writing is difficult for many researchers, even seniors. Hence, enough time should be reserved for this cumbersome exercise. It is also important to make sure well in advance that all the key members of the team are free and available to write their shares and review the manuscript(s) once the project has advanced to this point.

When working out the time schedule of the project, it is prudent to always anticipate complications whose exact nature may be unknown at that stage. They tend to be a rule rather than an exception. A technician may quit just when he or she has been fully trained and when the interobserver error has been recorded, the interviewer becomes pregnant in the middle of the project when everything else runs according to the schedule, the statistician suffers a heart attack 2 weeks before the data analysis, the pathologist who agreed to check the cancer diagnoses suddenly leaves for a 1-year assignment with the International Agency for Research on Cancer in Lyons, the delivery of necessary new equipment is 3 months delayed (and does not work even then), and so forth. Just when the report should be compiled (the deadline for the funding agency is coming up in 1 month!), the director of the institute decides to take a sabbatical leave and the main investigator must function as his stand-in. Not all of there, of course, will happen each time in each project, but it is very common that something similar or something even more unexpected occurs in every major project spanning over several years. One should therefore always make an allowance of half a year or more for unexpected complications.

Unexpected practical matters almost always disrupt the original time schedule.

The *project organization* should be decided at the planning stage. Who is responsible for what? Are the superiors of all team members truly committed? Have all the consultants (hygienists, statisticians, clinicians, etc.) really agreed to contribute? The roles and responsibilities of the various organizations and persons should be agreed upon and listed in sufficient detail.

The last but not least important part of the study plan is the *budget*. Realization of how expensive the ideal project would be often comes as the moment of truth for the overoptimistic researcher. If all real costs are considered, including the salaries of the regular staff, it can be a shocking to realize how expensive the planned project turns out to be. One should accept the fact that also one's own institution, not only the funding agency, must agree to the budget.

At this stage, if not before, the researcher must learn how to *set priorities*. Sometimes many measurements can (or must) be omitted, and the researcher must scrutinize the envisaged study material and decide whether it is too large. At this stage it is often necessary to lower the level of ambition (experienced epidemiologists have learned to do this at a much earlier stage). Late-stage revisions dictated by harsh economic realities frequently change the initial study plan, which then has to be revised downward.

Economic restrictions may force one to lower the ambition level of the project. This should be realized already at an early stage of the planning process.

Technically, the expenses must be specified as regular salaries (paid by the parent organization), salaries for temporary staff, costs of training the personnel, consultants, fees, social security payments, possible fees to examinees, costs of statistical and data services, equipment, laboratory, office and other supplies, costs of tracing drop-outs, mailing costs, fieldwork costs, costs of domestic and international travel, and publication costs. Sometimes office space and utilities must also be budgeted. It is also important to adjust the flow of payment to fit the respective stages of the project. If funding comes from a number of different sources, the tentative share of each one shall be specified. Experience has shown that the situation is easier to handle if only one funding agency is involved, but very large projects may require more than one source of funding.

PILOT STUDY

Sometimes so much uncertainty is involved in the planning of a large project that it is difficult or even impossible to envisage everything in advance. For example, it may be impossible to surmise if or to what extent the exposed subjects and especially the referents are willing to undergo medical examinations. It may also be hard to tell in advance whether the planned questionnaire is unambiguous and understandable to all. If the study population represents several linguistic groups, for example, English and Spanish speakers in the United States, or if there is a high percentage of guest workers of several nationalities in Europe, or if there are dozens of native languages, as in India, how should the questionnaire be administered? Are the translations quite identical and how should one handle illiterates? Would, after all, an interview be a better (although more expensive) alternative? If intervention is planned, how many subjects will volunteer, and how many will remain in the study after a certain period of time? What is the best way to motivate the participants? These and other questions may be impossible to answer before one knows how the program works in practice. In such situations a pilot study can determine if the project will succeed or not. The main purpose of the pilot study is to test the *feasibility* of the study procedure and the intended methods—not the advance testing of the study hypothesis on minimaterial.

A pilot study tests the feasibility of the project and attempts to improve its methods. It is not an advance test of the study hypothesis on minimaterial.

As a result of the pilot study, the choice of methods may change, the procedures for gathering material may turn out to be different from the initial ideas, and even the aim of the study may sometimes be modified. If this happens, the "results" gathered from the pilot study cannot be combined with those of the study proper, but as already pointed out, obtaining "results" is definitely not the aim of the pilot study. Its purpose is to solve practical problems related to the feasibility of the main project and to improve its quality.

Procedurewise, the pilot study can have been completed when the study plan is being submitted to the funding agency, or it can be the first phase of the plan, in which case reservations must be made for revision of the study plan later. Should the pilot study be part of the study plan proper or not, depends on whether special funding is needed for it. If there are any doubts about the feasibility of a large project, for example, an intervention, most reviewers of grant applications prefer to see the results of a pilot study before recommending funding.

PROJECT DIARY

When the study plan has been approved by the parent institution, or funding has been granted, the project is ready to start. This does not mean that the study plan can be filed and forgotten, and that everything from that point on will happen intuitively. The original plan should, in principle, be followed (otherwise it would be fraud), but because many things do not proceed as planned, some changes may have to be undertaken. Everything that happens during the course of the project should be put down in a *project diary*. This diary, together with the approved plan, can nowadays easily be set up in the form of a computer file. Such a file not only helps the main investigator to keep track of the scientific realization of the operational plan of the project, but also of its administrative and economic aspects.

Changes in the original plan were already referred to; it is also important to explain why they were done. There may be problems with access to the material, with data acquisition, with calibration of instruments, with running the analyses, and even with incompetence of members of the research team and the technicians. For example, the dates of employing new sets of reagents, the time of service of equipment, and the personnel's sick leaves and other leaves of absence should all be recorded. If blinding of readings is done, the code of identification is crucial. It should be made secret by means of code words so that those team members who must be blinded do not have access to it. There may be changes in the original data processing program and some measurements may be so absurd that they must be judged wrong. All this must be documented. All the crude measuring results should, of course, be recorded, and preliminary tables, even ones that are not intended to be published, may be constructed and kept in the computer files or a more conventional diary. The same is true for records of quality control of the methods, and all the scientifically less important data that are not going to be included in the publication. Detailed notes are of great help when the research report is drafted, when difficult letters from colleagues have to be answered, and when scientists visiting one's institution request specific data on procedural matters.

PUBLICATION

No research project is finished until it is published. Writing the report is hard work for many researchers, who would prefer to start their next study immediately. However, writing need not be that cumbersome. If the study plan is detailed and otherwise good, almost half of the report is already written. Working in an organized manner helps one avoid the chaotic stage so typical of the last months of many projects, when the researchers use weeks or months to sort out what on earth they should do with half a mile of computer write-outs, when they do not recall the reason why only half of the subjects showed up 2 years ago, or when they have no way of finding out anymore what the roentgenologic criteria were for the diagnosis of lung fibrosis, long forgotten by the radiologist who, besides, has recently moved to Hawaii and no longer replies to letters.

During a long project new literature usually accrues. This may influence the interpretation of the results of the project. If the literature surveillance has been systematic and continuous, the researcher is up to date and there is no fear of late-stage discoveries revealing that the study had been done on quite wrong premises.

All this should have been documented in the study protocol. If this has been the case, the researcher can concentrate on writing a good article without being hindered by logistic problems. Sometimes it may be difficult to extract the really essential findings from a vast amount of data. This is a test of maturity. Here, again, it is worthwhile to go back to the study plan and to recall what exactly the objectives were. The results providing answers to the primary questions are the vital ones. Less central results must be deleted from the main report because they only confuse its message; it may sometimes be justified to publish them later as by-products. Important observations and conclusions must not be hidden in a jungle of less weighty data.

Concentrate on relevant results; do not publish everything—that would only reveal your lack of discrimination.

The "discussion" section is the final maturity test of the researcher's insight and competence. It is here that the most central findings should be put into perspective, that the evidence supporting and contradicting the literature can be given, and where one can analyze any possible sources of error that may have distorted the author's own study (and earlier studies for that matter). Finally, the "discussion" should give the author's interpretation of the meaning of the present results.

Many good books have been published on how to write scientific articles. My favorite is Day's[1] book, which is easy to read, simple, and therefore excellent, although it deals mostly with experimental science (not only medicine). However, there are many others. Each junior researcher (and many seniors also) should read at least a couple of them. All the books I have read stress the importance of simplicity, brevity, and clarity. In epidemiologic articles, but perhaps also in others, the only exception to the rule of brevity is the "Material and Methods" section. This must be sufficiently detailed because of the many snags involved in epidemiologic research. The peer reviewers and all the other readers must be given the possibility to form their own opinion of the validity of the research.

Strive for brevity and clarity, but give enough details on materials and methods.

The language should be simple, because many of the potential readers are not native English speakers. The main purpose of an article is to convey a message, not to show how eloquent the author is. British authors, in particular, sometimes use language that is difficult even for American readers, not to mention of others. One should avoid technical jargon (words or expressions understandable only for those working in the same narrow field). Authors whose native language is not English should always have their draft revised by a competent *native* linguistic reviewer (the American-born language editor of the journal I am editing firmly holds that this also applies to most native speakers of English).

Remember that most of your readers are not native English speakers. Be simple, use easy language, and avoid jargon. Ask a linguistic expert to check your manuscript, even if you are a native English speaker.

Formal matters, such as compliance with the "Instructions for Authors," good concise language, neat typing, good quality figures, and, for example, the German, Italian, and French names correctly spelled in the reference list, mean more than most authors realize, especially when the editor's desk is covered by huge piles of manuscripts, only a third or less of which can find space in the journal. It is also wise to ask for comments from colleagues before submitting the article to a journal, because there are many kinds of "blinding" in science, among them the inability to see one's own mistakes.

As Day[1] states, a scientific article is the researcher's visiting card. The quality of the researcher's writing is decisive for his or her professional reputation in the scientific world, not how nice a chap he is or how funny are the jokes she tells at congress dinners. Therefore the importance of thoroughly polishing any written contribution cannot be stressed too much.

REFERENCES

1. Day, R.A. *How to Write and Publish a Scientific Paper* (ISI Press, Philadelphia, PA, 1979).
2. Miettinen, O. S. *Theoretical Epidemiology: Principles of Occurrence Research in Medicine* (New York: John Wiley & Sons, 1985).

CHAPTER 8

Ethical Aspects

Although ethical problems are usually characteristic of clinical and experimental studies, epidemiologic investigations are not free from them. Epidemiologists have only lately become aware of these aspects.

Epidemiologic research often utilizes data from computerized registers. Access to such data is usually regulated by legislation that protects their privacy. Due to the long time span of many epidemiologic studies, both the data obtained from registers and those gathered directly from the study population, may have to be stored for long periods of time. The personal data must be protected during the entire period and they must be properly destroyed when the study has been completed. Moreover, epidemiologic studies deal with people of whom the majority are "healthy," at least at the beginning of the study period. Subjecting such persons to clinical examinations presents problems that are very different from those encountered in clinical research on sick patients, who may benefit from many of the examinations. Questionnaire studies often inquire into matters that can be experienced as sensitive; care must be taken not to hurt the feelings of the subject.

In the following, some central ethical aspects are discussed. They have been selected mostly because of their general character. Each single study may, in addition, have specific problems.

The study must be carried out in *the best possible way*. Poorly planned and conducted research is always unethical. Wrong conclusions drawn from a poor study can result in considerable human suffering or economic losses (e.g., because a carcinogen escapes identification, because redesign of a workplace is done on wrong grounds, because different hygienic improvements are given wrong priorities). The results of the study must always be made available to the community. This usually calls for publication in a scientific or at least a professional journal. Failing to publish the results means that the examinees have been abused and the funding has been wasted. The researchers themselves undoubtedly intend to publish their results when starting the project (why should they do research otherwise?), but, especially if the results are not very "exciting" or if a central member leaves the team, the writing of the report may just be left undone. Sometimes someone else may try to prevent or at least delay publication. It may be the management (if the research is done in a company), superiors in a research institute having "internal peer review," or even outsiders, such as labor market organizations or industrial companies. Typical arguments are that the results are inconclusive, that there are methodologic errors or that "further research" must first be carried out. This is not to say that errors in execution of the study or interpretation of the results should not be corrected, but since no epidemiologic study is perfect, such arguments can easily be abused. Censorship is always unethical, unless the reason is a major flaw in the study. Minor errors are not a sufficient reason for rejection, provided the authors discuss them openly.

The results should be published in such a form and language that they are understandable to the different target groups. This often requires two or more levels of reporting, one scientific and one popular. Moreover, the study protocols and the raw data should be kept for many years in order to allow other epidemiologists to check the details of the study, if needed, and to replicate the investigation.

The *interpretation* of the results must be objective. All the relevant literature must be reviewed, not only those articles that fit in with the researchers' own view. All pertinent data must be shown, not only "suitable" ones. Errors must be pinpointed, and validity problems discussed openly. Creating sensations in the news media is not the proper way for serious researchers to communicate with the public, especially if the results are uncertain.

Research contracts must be strictly complied with, with regard to adherence to the study protocol, the confidentiality of individual measurements, the publication scheme, and the use of funds. One should never sign contracts limiting the right to free, scientific publication. Unfortunately, studies done within companies are not always guaranteed free scientific publication (and many are never published). When signing a research contract, one should also agree in advance on how the news media are to be informed, and whose responsibility that will be.

Information on the objectives of the study and how it will be carried out must be given to everybody involved. Depending on the source of information, written study descriptions may be required for registers, companies, unions, and authorities. Personal information is required whenever the study involves measurements carried out on individuals. Enough information should also be given to the workplaces involved so that everyone concerned knows what is going on. The participants must be told exactly what medical examinations will be done and their purpose should be explained. The full consent of the participants is obligatory. Everyone must have the freedom to decide whether or not to participate. The right of participants' to know what the study may reveal is regulated by law in some countries. All participants should be given their individual results, preferably with recommendations on what to do (e.g., "everything is all right," "contact your doctor," and so forth). If agreed in advance, the results can alternatively be given directly to the worker's plant physician or family doctor. However, otherwise, they are confidential, meaning, for example, that the management cannot be informed.

Examinations that may pose some *risk* or that are *painful* or *unpleasant* are usually considered unethical. For example, because of the radiation risk involved, roentgenologic examinations are nowadays often considered unethical in cohort or cross-sectional studies, in which most of the subjects are healthy with respect to the disease of interest. On the other hand, a roentgenologic examination of, say, the lumbar spine may be quite well motivated in a case-referent study because the "case" is ill and may benefit from such an examination. In the Nordic countries blood sampling is considered acceptable, whereas in some other countries this procedure is considered too painful (or unethical for religious reasons). If blood samples are taken, tests other than those agreed upon between the parties involved should not be done. "Extra" tests that may hurt the integrity of the subject (e.g., blood alcohol, human immunodeficiency virus antibodies, drug metabolites) can under no circumstances be considered ethical without the subject's special permission. Often these and other restrictions, especially the requirement of freedom from risk for the subject, restrict the choice of examinations suitable for epidemiologic studies as compared with those available for clinical studies.

If, in the course of a prospective study, it becomes evident that individual exposure levels *exceed safe limits*, the researcher must take the initiative to remove the subject from the hazardous exposure, even at the cost of loss of information (see Chapter 4, Example 8). The decision lies with the employer, not the researchers, but the latter must inform the employer's representative and give their own recommendation. Likewise, if a cross-sectional study reveals health hazards, the researchers must act so that everyone concerned receives correct and sufficient information to enable preventive action.

In occupational health research any intervention must be in the direction of *reducing or eliminating harmful exposure*. If some exposing agent is substituted by another, there must be guarantees that the new agent is less harmful than the original one. If the intervention entails the termination of the exposure by transferring workers to jobs without exposure, the new task must not hurt the workers economically by causing reductions in income or other benefits. Interventions necessitating increased physical exercise, for example, for the sake of preventing back disorders, must be so designed that persons with other ailments, for example, heart conditions, do not suffer harm from them. Sometimes a health examination is needed to exclude risk individuals before enrolling subjects to the program. The results of such examinations must not be used to endanger the continuation of the worker's employment.

Interventions made in the occupational health setting generally pose less ethical problems than clinical trials because of the requirement that the intervention must be in the direction of reducing exposure.

Sensitive items are sometimes included in questionnaires and interviews. It is important to consider thoroughly what questions really are needed and what information is less important. For instance, information on the use of alcohol may be central in a study on the effects of solvent exposure on primary liver cancer incidence, but unnecessary when the effects of foundry work on the incidence of bronchitis are studied. Questions pertaining to neuroticism are relevant in a study of work stress, but inappropriate if the issue is the connection between pesticide exposure and soft tissue sarcoma.

The interviewer must always be considerate, tactful, patient, friendly, and empathetic. The interview must proceed logically and be adjusted to the intellectual capacity of the person interviewed. The interviewer must show respect to those interviewed, irrespective of how they behave. The interview should not be too exhaustive, especially when sick people are being interviewed. These requirements are stringent and disqualify many people from becoming interviewers. Even interviewers with good personal qualifications require thorough training.

Interviewing the *close relatives of deceased persons* is usually a delicate task that requires utmost tact and consideration. If possible, the interview should be postponed until the mourning process is over. This process usually takes 1 year, on average. Interviewing even many years later may recall painful memories, hence, tact is always needed. Also the interviewing of the close relatives of severely ill persons, for example, parents of children suffering from cancer, is very demanding. The relatives themselves can also be physically or mentally ill, especially the next-of-kin of deceased old persons. The interviewer may not be aware of their health state beforehand and caution is therefore important.

Confidentiality requirements must always be adhered to. No individual data can be revealed to outsiders, for example, to employers. Also the confidential nature of data gathered from registers and data bases must be taken into consideration. The right of individual companies to keep their conditions confidential (e.g., the results of hygienic measurements) must be respected. Most countries have a data protection law and also special legislation concerning medical records, social security benefits, and employers' registers. In some countries (e.g., France and Germany) the legislation is so strict that cohort mortality studies are nearly impossible to carry out.

From an ethical point of view, the *reference group* is even more problematic than the study group. The reason is that most subjects themselves rarely benefit from serving as referents. If the study involves clinical examinations, one could therefore consider adding some extra tests to the scheme for the reference group. These may not be so relevant from the point of view of the study objectives, but they could provide the reference subjects with useful information on their own health state and thereby make the study more meaningful to them. Examples of such extra tests that are painless, pose no risk, and can be of benefit for the subjects, in addition to being rather inexpensive, are blood pressure measurements, electrocardiography, and some simple blood chemistry, if blood samples are taken anyway. Such examinations could be included if there are available funds.

Questionnaire and interview studies, in which the study hypothesis cannot be revealed for the sake of avoiding information bias, can be ethically problematic. One should also remember that some patients are not aware of the true nature of their disease, perhaps because their physician has felt that they would not be able to cope with the information. It would be a grave mistake to reveal serious diagnoses in an interview or questionnaire study (e.g., by beginning the session by stating that "you have been chosen to this study because you have cancer''). Specific diseases should therefore not be mentioned. If the interview takes place in a hospital in connection with the normal hospital routine, the patient usually experiences the situation as less annoying than when a complete stranger suddenly rings the doorbell or telephones home.

The research must be *honest*. It is sad that one has to state this self-evident matter in a text like this one, but there have been several examples of fraudulent research during the last 10 years or so.[1] It is considered dishonest to manipulate the data, to apply wrong methods of data collection or analysis, to withhold part of the evidence, or to misinterpret it deliberately. Inventing data is, of course, also dishonest, but because epidemiologic studies usually represent teamwork, the prospects of getting away with this type of fraud are poor. If epidemiologists find themselves in situations where the interests of the parties involved are in conflict (e.g., unions vs employers), an impartial expert role must be maintained.

Recently, it has become more common for epidemiologists to appear in a court of law, for example, in matters related to legal compensation for possible occupational diseases, or in hearings, for example, when new proposals for standards or norms are being tried. This is a very complicated matter. As long as the epidemiologist remains honest, this practice can be justified. However, usually the epidemiologist represents one of the parties and impartiality is then not possible. There have been many examples of misconduct in such situations, the worst probably being systematic discrediting of others' research by magnifying the errors that always can be found from epidemiologic studies. One-sided interpretation of scientific data is another example.

In summary, the researcher must ensure that the study does not hurt the subjects in any way, be it physical, psychological, or economic. The subjects must be fully informed about the objectives and methods of the study, their participation must be voluntary, and they must be informed of their personal test results. Bad science is always unethical. Nowadays there are ethical committees in most institutions and their approval must be sought before any project can start. This gives at least some guarantees for ethical research. However, there is nothing that prevents epidemiologists from ''prostituting'' themselves in courts and hearings.

REFERENCES

1. Smith, J. ''Preventing fraud,'' *Br. Med. J.* 302:362 (1991).

CHAPTER 9

Some Guidelines for Interpreting Epidemiologic Studies

INTRODUCTION

The result of an epidemiologic study can reflect a true relation, be due to chance, or be biased. The researcher should be able to evaluate how "true" the achieved result is. In addition, the reader of the researcher's report should be able to judge which alternative is the most likely one. This chapter offers some guidelines for the critical evaluation of epidemiologic study results.

Interpretation of a study goes beyond merely checking if the results are "correct." In science the ultimate goal is to move from the particular to the abstract-general. Hence the experience gained from the study is not interesting as such. It should only be regarded as a means of complementing or changing one's abstract view of the nature of matters.[5]

The interpretation of a single study relies heavily on individual judgment. Experts may disagree on whether the results of the study are valid or not, on their meaning, not to speak of the scientific generalizations they may lead to. Therefore, the authors of an article should be careful not to serve the readers their own views as the only truth; instead they must give the readers a fair chance to form their own, independent judgment. This opportunity is best created by giving the readers access to the same relevant data that underlied the authors' conclusions. Hence it is important that the article presents the pertinent details, in addition to being concisely and well written.

A person's posterior view is composed of that person's prior view and the comparatively small amount of new information a particular study may have produced. This is the very reason why the synthesis of data is subjective; the prior view is by far the largest component of a posteriori knowledge. It is well known that experts often disagree on scientific matters although their information comes from the same published sources. Therefore two or more parallel views often prevail, and, contrary to what is often believed, these "prevailing views" are subjective, because they are formed from judgments and syntheses made by human beings.

It goes without saying that thorough insight into the subject matter is necessary for any competent interpretation of a study. Almost equally important is the understanding of epidemiologic principles and of scientific inference in general. However, mere understanding of epidemiologic methodology, even though extremely important, is not enough for going beyond a purely technical evaluation of what is correct and what is incorrect in a particular study. If the reader's prior view of the scientific issue is incomplete and confused, the posterior view will also be unclear, in spite of perfect technical evaluation of the article in question.

According to conventional statistical thinking, the results of a particular study should be interpreted independently of prior knowledge, in other words, without letting earlier knowledge influence one's conclusions on whether the results are "correct" or not. No one would ignore previous experience in the decision-making of everyday life. Why should one do so in science?

Bayesian thinking offers an alternative to the conventional "frequentist" view. Bayes was a clergyman and mathematician who lived in the 18th century. He studied conditional probabilities and formulated a theorem describing their relationships. The essence of Bayes' theorem, when applied to epidemiology, is that the posterior credibility, or odds, of the study hypothesis being correct is the product of the prior odds and the likelihood ratio. In other words,

$$\text{Posterior odds} = \text{prior odds} \times \text{likelihood ratio}$$

In general, the likelihood ratio is the ratio of the probabilities that an observed association is consistent with either the study (alternative) hypothesis (H_A) or the null hypothesis (H_0). Hence,

$$LR = \frac{P \text{ (observed association}|H_A)}{P \text{ (observed association}|H_0)}$$

where P means probability and | denotes "conditional on."

The problem with Bayesian statistics is the difficulty to define prior credibility, especially that of no prior information. Prior credibility depends on the synthesis of all available evidence, whether it be epidemiologic, experimental, or theoretical, and the outcome of such a synthesis is subjective. In addition, the computation of posterior credibility is often complicated, especially if many parameters are involved.

Bayesian thinking is different from the "frequentist" approach, according to which the outcome of a particular study is tested and evaluated irrespective of previous studies. However, no rationally thinking scientist would ignore all that is known from before and make his or her interpretation of a scientific study merely on the basis of that study. As Miettinen[5] states: ". . . the documented evidence does not represent the ultimate *result* of the study. As the objective is to learn about *abstract* quantities and relations, the actual result of the study could be taken as the *view* about the abstract object of the study that the study leads to, or as the change in the *view* brought about by the study" (p. 107). If one agrees with this statement, then a "result" means far more than a statistically significant difference obtained from a set of data.

The "prevailing view" is usually subjective in science.

CHECKING VALIDITY

The reader cannot evaluate a study unless the authors have described its design, materials, and methods in sufficient detail. In fact, the materials and methods section should be so detailed that another competent researcher could replicate the study from the author's description (see Chapter 7). If the article contains only superficial, incomplete, or otherwise poor descriptions of the materials and the methods, the reader cannot escape the impression that the authors are nonchalant or incompetent or both. Sometimes the authors may even avoid going into detail on purpose for the very reason that they realize that the study has flaws. Irrespective of the reason for deficient reporting, such articles are scientifically uninformative.

The reader can evaluate a study only if the researchers give sufficiently detailed descriptions of its design, materials, and methods.

In general, readers neither have the time nor the reason to scrutinize every article very thoroughly. Most people read only the abstract. However, under certain circumstances, the scientific literature must be analyzed in great detail. Thorough reading is required, for example, when one is compiling the scientific basis needed to establish hygienic standards and other regulations. In addition, the classification of chemicals into different categories of carcinogenicity can only be done after careful scrutiny of all pertinent articles. The acceptance of papers to be published in scientific journals is highly dependent on the recommendations given by the scientific referees of the manuscripts. Such peer review also presupposes thorough reading. When such critical evaluations are being made, for whatever reason, it is useful to proceed in an orderly fashion (cf. also Chapter 7). The following guidelines should help readers achieve a systematic approach to a scientific article:

1. One should note who the *authors* are and from what institution the article comes. Researchers are, unfortunately, not equal; a good scientific reputation offers some (although not complete) guarantee that the study is sound.

2. The *study design* should be appropriate and efficient. Crude register linkage studies, for example, are less conclusive than detailed cohort studies. Case-referent studies are inefficient when the exposure is rare in the base, and the same is true for cohort studies if the outcome is rare.

3. Although long reviews of the literature are not recommended nowadays, the reader should make sure that the authors have referred to the literature in a balanced way. Balanced does not mean that all weak articles must be mentioned, but there should be reference to views that are in conflict with those of the authors, if such literature exists.

4. The *objectives* of the study should be clearly stated, and it should be easy to check if the authors have succeeded in achieving them. It is important to distinguish between a qualitative and a quantitative study, and one should make sure that the authors have realized this.

5. The reader must be able to judge what *prior hypothesis* the study was designed to test, or whether the study was explorative only. Was the hypothesis so formulated that it was testable?

6. The *materials and methods* section should contain a clear definition of the study base. The article must state how common the phenomenon under study was in that base. From this information, the reader can judge whether the sample size was sufficient. There should be thorough descriptions of the exposed and reference groups (Chapter 7). One should especially consider whether the sample was representative of the category it should represent (Chapter 5). If the general population was the reference category, the reasons, if any, should be stated. How much did this choice weaken the inference made from the study?

7. The methods of *data collection* should be so well described that the reader can pinpoint flaws, if there are any. In addition the measurement methods, the criteria for abnormality, and other diagnostic criteria should be clearly stated.

8. The *validity* of the study must be evaluated. The reader should be provided with enough information to check the comparability of the examined groups, for example, how the subjects were selected into the study and remained there, if the information was symmetric, if the methods were controlled and how, and what the methods were for controlling confounding. The possibility of nondifferential misclassification should be considered in studies with negative results.

9. The *statistical analysis* must be correct. Medical readers usually need the advice of a competent statistician for this evaluation. Equally important is an insightful interpretation of the tests. Too much reliance on mere p-values does not indicate scientific insight.

10. It is important to consider whether the main results are in concordance or in conflict with the *prevailing view* (or with which one of them, if there are several). If they are conflicting, what could the reason be?

11. Finally, the reader should judge how the authors *interpret* their results. Are their conclusions sound or too far-reaching? Is it possible to agree with the authors' reasoning.

Even if systematic errors have not been totally controlled, the study may not necessarily be a complete failure. It is important to consider the direction and strength of such errors. Minor bias does not necessarily invalidate a study, especially if its quantitative effect can be evaluated. One should remember that confounding and other systematic errors are not always effect magnifying, as many people seem to think. They can equally well mask or reduce a true effect. Good epidemiologists usually point out possible errors in their studies and discuss the effects of them. Very often a study can give useful information in spite of some minor invalidity.

Generalization requires the internal validity to be at least reasonable; otherwise the study is meaningless. One should clearly distinguish between the particularistic sample-to-population generalization, which is done from the results of descriptive surveys, and the scientific generalization to the abstract-general, which is the aim of etiologic studies. Results that may modify prevailing views are especially interesting, but the search for alternative explanations (bias, random errors) must be more intense than usual, because of the low prior credibility of the result.

STATISTICAL SIGNIFICANCE

Statistical significance has been referred to many times and the p-value was briefly presented in Chapter 5. In this context some guidelines for the interpretation of statistical significance are given.

Significance testing is applied to assess formally the likelihood that the result of a comparison either complies with the study hypothesis or its denial, the null hypothesis. This probability is usually summarized as the p-value. It is conventionally said that, under the null hypothesis (i.e., provided no true effect indeed exists), the p-value expresses the probability of the "true" difference being more extreme than the one found. However, the magnitude of the difference is not formulated in any study hypothesis; moreover, the same difference gives a low p-value in a large material and a higher p-value in a small material. Using conventional language, one can say that the same result would have been "significant" for a large material and "nonsignificant" for a small one. Therefore, not only the magnitude of the difference, but also the amount of information in the data, determine the p-value (see Chapter 5).

If the material is small, the point estimate of the RR varies randomly within wide limits, and the p-value also contains little information. Such a study is uninformative. If, on the other hand, the material is very large, even a minimal difference gives a very small p-value. Such a small difference is without biological meaning. Besides, such a difference can easily arise from undetected slight confounding or some other bias. Therefore, in very large studies, the p-value alone does not convey much information. One can say that the p-value is too sensitive to be useful in very large studies. Such results should rather be analyzed quantitatively by interval estimation than qualitatively only by significance testing.

Example 1. Suppose that the cumulative mortality is 10% in a follow-up study comprising 1000 exposed subjects and 1000 referents. Then $\widehat{RR}$ = 1.5 is statistically significant (p = 0.01). The same level of significance requires $\widehat{RR}$ = 11 in a study comprising only 50 exposed and 50 unexposed subjects. Let us further suppose that the issue is the effect of chromate exposure on lung cancer. From Tables 2 and 3 (Chapter 5) it can be seen that confounding by smoking could explain the $\widehat{RR}$ of the larger study. By contrast, an undetected confounding of sufficient strength to cause a confounded $\widehat{RR}$ of 11 would not be possible. $\widehat{RR}$ = 1.5 would have been far from significant in the smaller study, and $\widehat{RR}$ = 11 would, of course, have been very convincingly significant in the large study. In the small study, the $\widehat{RR}$ = 11 does not convey much quantitative information because of the wide confidence interval, while the $\widehat{RR}$ = 1.5 of the large study is so stable that one also can assess the strength of the effect in quantitative terms.

The p-value can best be interpreted in medium-sized studies. Biologically insignificant differences do not give low p-values and the random variation of the estimate of the RR is reasonable. Moreover, slight invalidity does not cause very small p-values. A very small p-value obtained from a medium-sized study is more compatible with the study hypothesis than with its denial; it intuitively supports the study hypothesis. A small p-value (say, 0.10 to 0.20) is devoid of meaning because it does not discriminate between the null hypothesis and the study hypothesis, while an intermediate or a large p-value supports the null hypothesis. The expression "intuitively" is used on purpose because there are no precise definitions for terms like "large," "small," and "very small." This is true both for the amount of information (the size of the study and how common the phenomenon is), and for the numerical value of p. Commonly used borders of significance (e.g., 0.05) are arbitrary, as discussed in Chapter 5. The malpractice of mechanically "accepting" or "rejecting" the study hypothesis (or the null hypothesis, for that sake) merely on whether p < 0.05 or p > 0.05, as unfortunately is often done, reveals lack of scientific insight.

The high sensitivity of p-values derived from large studies should, of course, not lead one to discharge such information as being unimportant. On the contrary, large studies give reliable quantitative estimates of the true RR because its estimate is more stable, the larger the study. Therefore, in large studies, the $\widehat{RR}$ and its confidence interval, not the p-value, convey the relevant information. Hence, especially in this situation, interval estimation should be applied rather than qualitative hypothesis testing.

In large studies, the estimate of the rate ratio is informative, while the p-value is not. In intermediate-sized studies, the p-value is informative. In small studies, both are uninformative.

Several alternatives exist, as a rule, for the statistical analysis of the data. Usually researchers, or rather their statistical consultants, prefer tests having the best power to discriminate between the study hypothesis and the null hypothesis. Unfortunately, wrong tests are sometimes used, tests whose assumptions are not fulfilled in the data. Moreover, the reader must be able to judge if correct statistics have been applied. Therefore the statistic from which the p-value was derived must be given, not merely the p-value, or even worse, only an indication that the result was "significant." In addition, the author should mention whether a *one-* or *two-sided test* has been used. A one-sided test assumes that the effect can have one direction only, while a two-sided test assesses both causative and preventive effects. Usually two-sided tests are used indiscriminately. An etiologic hypothesis very rarely has two directions; it would be like postulating that an exposure is *either* harmful *or* preventive. Most causal hypotheses take the form that exposure A causes disease B or that disease B is caused by exposures A and C (see Chapter 1). Preventive hypotheses state that exposure A (e.g., a diet) prevents disease B or that a reduction in exposure C prevents disease B. These are clearly unidirectional hypotheses, and therefore testing their counterparts by computing two-sided p-values makes little sense. A two-sided test should, on the other hand, be used in clinical trials because usually there is no certain prior evidence that the new treatment is more efficient than the conventional one. Two-sided tests should also be used in so-called "explorative" studies without prior hypothesis.

One-sided tests are usually appropriate in occupational epidemiology because this discipline investigates etiologic hypotheses, according to which the biological effect has one direction only (e.g., asbestos exposure causes bronchial carcinoma). p-Values from one-sided tests are usually considered to be twice as "sensitive" as the corresponding values from two-sided tests, the latter of the two generally being given in statistical tables. A one-sided p-value can be obtained by simply dividing the two-sided p-value listed in such a table by two. However, when one decides in favor of one-sided hypothesis testing, it is important that the observed difference is in the hypothesized direction. Otherwise the one-sided p-value would be misleading. If the data show, for example, a protective instead of a harmful effect, it is better not to give any p-value at all, only to state that the result was not in the expected direction. Of course the interpretation of a study should not rely too much on whether some arbitrary level of significance has been achieved or not. However, using a one-sided p-value instead of a two-sided value can formally change a "nonsignificant" result into a "significant" one (e.g., $p = 0.03$ instead of 0.06). Researchers with insight into epidemiology do not dichotomize in such a manner. But there are many kinds of readers of epidemiologic studies. As long as statistical significance is considered so central for scientific judgment, the author should at least provide the reader with the right type of p-value. However, the term "statistically significant" could well be abandoned in epidemiologic writing. Instead of using this cliché, the authors should mention the statistic used, then give the exact p-value, and finally state whether it is one- or two-sided. This system would leave the judgment of how "significant" the result is to each individual reader.

One-sided p-values are appropriate for testing unidirectional hypotheses.

As already stated, in occupational epidemiology quantitative interval estimation is usually to be preferred over qualitative hypothesis testing. Furthermore, in the presence of systematic errors, such as the healthy worker effect, significance testing is meaningless. It may even be misleading if interpreted uncritically. This problem arises especially when the mortality of an exposed cohort is being compared to that of the general population (Chapter 5). Such results should not be expressed in terms of statistical significance; unfortunately, such terms are still being used all too often. The confidence interval for the estimate of the SMR gives better information. It shows within what limits the true parameter is likely to be located without falsely implying that a "significant" or "nonsignificant" result has been obtained from a comparison that was valid, which is the impression a p-value can give unlearned readers.

According to conventional "frequentist" statistical thinking, the interpretation of the data must take into account the number of comparisons made simultaneously. By definition, one out of twenty test results is "significant" at the 5% level. If enough comparisons are made, some tests will automatically be significant without having any biologic meaning, so the saying goes. The constellation of many simultaneous comparisons, giving rise to several "significant" p-values, is called the *multisignificance phenomenon*. Formally, with this way of thinking one can say that if n independent associations are tested for statistical significance, the chance that at least one of them will turn out "significant" is $1 - (1 - alpha)^n$, on the presumtion that all null hypotheses are true. This way of reasoning implies that there is a "universal" null hypothesis according to which nothing is interrelated. Such thinking is definitely not supported by empirical science.[10] It must be quite evident that, from the point of view of one particular hypothesis, it is totally irrelevant how many other unrelated comparisons are being made at the same time.[5] For example, for testing the hypothesis that benzene exposure causes leukemia (and supposing that a positive association is found), it is absolutely irrelevant if twenty, ten, or no other chemicals are investigated in the same study. It is the credibility of the prior hypothesis that matters, not the number of comparisons. However, if the hypotheses are related, the situation is different; such hypotheses must be examined jointly. For example, if lead exposure slows the conduction velocity in one nerve, it probably does so in others as well. Then the likelihood of finding at least one ''significant'' slowing increases, as the number of nerves being tested increases.

The statistical testing of a particular hypothesis is independent of how many other unrelated comparisons are being made from the same data.

On the other hand, if many comparisons are made in an explorative study without any prior hypothesis, a true multisignificance situation may arise. This constellation should be distinguished from a study that has primarily been designed to test a specific hypothesis, but in which the researcher, in addition, takes advantage of the additional data collected, to explore other associations as well. For example, linking a cancer register with occupational data from a census 10 years earlier is such an explorative study. However, even in this constellation some associations have higher prior credibility than others, and the interpretation cannot rely on mere p-values.

Conventional statistical thinking also distinguishes between the testing of prior hypotheses, meaning those which the investigators had in mind when initiating the study, and data-suggested hypotheses, meaning those new ones that came up when the data were at hand. One speaks about ''hypothesis-testing'' and ''hypothesis-generating'' studies. In the same spirit it is also claimed that data that were first used for hypothesis generation cannot be utilized in the testing of that hypothesis. In other words, one must use new material for that purpose. Bayesian epidemiologists disagree with this viewpoint.[5] Close adherence to these principles would harm epidemiologic research. Often a particular study, initiated to test a certain hypothesis, yields a large amount of secondary information on the same subjects. For example, a cohort study on the connection between arsenic exposure and lung cancer may also show an excess of some other cancer forms and of coronary heart disease, without any well-formulated prior hypotheses. Obviously few investigators would refrain from testing such results. Furthermore, when formally or informally evaluating all prior evidence, be it by a meta-analysis or intuitionally, hypothesis-generating and hypothesis-testing historical studies are almost never distinguished between. The evidence provided by the data is independent of anyone's knowledge before that person became aware of the data. If the prior credibility of the result obtained was low, the result itself will change that credibility only marginally. If, on the other hand, rethinking in the light of the new data reveals that the prior evidence was wrongly assessed, the revised prior credibility becomes higher, as does the posterior credibility.[5] However, experience shows that data-suggested hypotheses are usually wrong, whereas prior hypotheses are often correct.

Statistical testing presupposes absence of systematic errors. No significance test can discriminate between a true difference and one caused by bias. If the validity of the study is low, statistical testing is meaningless and misleading.

Statistical testing is meaningless and misleading in the presence of systematic errors.

POSITIVE AND NEGATIVE ERRORS

Systematic errors and wrong conclusions can either be in a positive or negative direction. Positivity/negativity is not an either–or matter, but a continuum. Results that, in fact, are slightly positive can, because they contain bias or because of misinterpretation, appear either intermediately or strongly positive or, conversely, as slightly or intermediately negative (''slightly'' negative can in this sense be thought of as not significantly deviating from unity, and ''intermediately'' as significantly less than unity, but not much). The common reasoning in terms of black and white probably comes from the bad habit of regarding results either as statistically significant (= positive) or nonsignificant (= negative), on the basis of arbitrary cut-off points for the p-value, and forgetting that systematic errors cannot be assessed by means of statistical significance testing. The continuous nature of the positivity/ negativity scale should be kept in mind as the following discussion on ''false positive'' and ''false negative'' results is read.

False Positive Results

The most common reasons for false positivity are, apart from chance, information bias and confounding; also selection bias can sometimes give a false positive result. Large studies can be misinterpreted if too much weight is given to statistical significance, because even minor bias can lead to small p-values. In smaller studies, statistical significance requires much larger differences. Therefore, should the difference be influenced by systematic errors, these errors must be so substantial that they are very evident.

In case-referent studies, the best known reason for false positive results is *information bias*. Information bias arises if the cases recall past events better than the referents or if the interviewer interviews the cases more intensively (see Chapter 5). It is usually assumed that information bias easily invalidates case-referent studies, being based, as they are, on anamnestic data. However, the strength of the information bias probably depends on the type of matters inquired into, rather than on some general rule (see Chapter 5). True, if such bias occurs, it is more likely to be positive than negative. However, in occupational epidemiology there is little empirical evidence of the occurrence of such bias, and, if recall is difficult, different types of matters are remembered in different detail.[1] This is not to say that the memory of interviewed people would be accurate — it is definitely not — but it is to say that the tendency for *asymmetrical* recall of cases and referents has not been convincingly shown empirically.

Selection bias can also cause false positive results in case-referent studies. Such errors can arise when the exposure under study influences the selection of cases and referents into the investigation. Case-referent studies on hospitalized patients can be especially problematic. In addition, the proneness to answer questionnaires or interviews can be different for cases and referents. If the response rates are much different, conclusions must be drawn with caution. The authors of the article should document in what respects those who responded differed from those who did not. Without having this type of information, the reader cannot evaluate the results. Errors caused by differences in the response rate can, of course, also be negative.

In cohort studies, *confounding* is probably a more important source of error than selection and information bias as far as false positive results are concerned. However, confounding usually has a negative direction, at least when occupational cohorts are being compared to the general population. Concomitant or earlier other occupational exposures may confound the study of work-related diseases even more than smoking and other life-style factors.

A *distorted or biased study base* can lead to a false positive conclusion. The study base is biased whenever it is unrepresentative of the study domain. Examples of this situation are outcome-dependent membership in the base population (see Example 2), outcome-dependent end of the follow-up (e.g., when "enough" cases have occurred), result-dependent deeper investigation of the data base (e.g., more thorough than average analysis of "interesting" findings), and result-dependent reporting (exciting positive results being submitted for publication and negative results never being reported).

Example 2. In a study of occupational liver disease, the basic material comprised 800 patients who had had a diagnostic liver biopsy.[11] Liver specimens were selected from those 23 patients who had been "exposed to chemicals" *and* referred to biopsy because of abnormally elevated liver function tests. Not surprisingly, the investigators found a variety of structural nonspecific abnormalities when they applied comprehensive and sophisticated methods of examination, such as electron microscopy. No proper reference group was used. The authors concluded that chemical exposure was the cause of the abnormalities found by the electron microscopy. It is clear that structural abnormalities *must* be found in a series of patients selected in this way. (Why was liver biopsy performed if not because of suspected liver disease?) Moreover, because the source material contained *both* subjects who had abnormal liver enzymes (the majority of them) *and* exposure to chemicals, it is inevitable that there were subjects having both attributes by mere coincidence. Hence, some of the "exposed" indeed also must have had structural abnormalities. Any occupational activity, even office work, can be incriminated as being hepatotoxic—and toxic to whatever target organ—if the study base is biased in such a manner.[4]

The *literature as a whole* can also be positively biased. This possibility has to do both with the earlier-mentioned result-dependent submittal of manuscripts to scientific journals and with the fact that editors, in general, indeed prefer positive findings over nonpositive ones. The human mind is such that positive findings feel more "exciting" than negative ones, and neither editors nor their referees are exceptions. The worst aspect of the publication bias is that especially so-called better journals succumb to this temptation, because of the very fact that they have a larger selection of manuscripts and a higher rejection rate than less prestigious periodicals. First reports of a phenomenon can be especially heavily biased in the positive direction because of these circumstances.

> *Example 3.* Consider a random cluster of congenital malformations occurring in a small group of female workers. Suppose also that the cluster turns out to be statistically significant ($p < 0.01$). Such a finding will easily reach the news media. This situation happened, in fact, some years ago. Small groups of women working at video terminals in different companies in North America gave birth to unexpectedly high numbers of babies with various congenital malformations. These results were mostly "published" in daily newspapers, but they caused quite a sensation. Several years later, no biological explanation has yet been found for why video terminal work would be teratogenic. In the United States alone, tens of such clusters of congenital malformations could be expected to occur in small groups by pure chance. Therefore, it is not surprising that somebody without insight, either in epidemiology or in teratology, can stumble on such a random cluster. The point is that such a finding should not be given a causal interpretation merely based on a statistically significant p-value, without the prior credibility of the finding being considered. No well-designed, sufficiently large epidemiologic study has so far (1991) been able to confirm these "findings." By contrast, the large number of studies published showing no effect, as well as the persistent lack of a biological explanation, have even added to the credibility of the view that there indeed is no effect.[6]

When a sufficient number of small groups are "exposed," it is possible that several similar results find their way into the literature and provide "supporting evidence." This development could lead to lower prior credibility for a negative study on the same topic. Truly negative results are difficult to produce because they require much larger materials, and, as a consequence, much more time and larger funds (see the next section). When even researchers regard positive results as more exciting than negative ones, it is no wonder that convincing the exposed workers and the general public of the absence of a risk can be hard, especially if there is so much published "evidence" supporting it. Uncritical conclusions drawn by some researchers from results that are technically correct, but may have quite other explanations, can indeed bias the literature in a positive direction.

First reports in the literature may be biased toward positivity.

Errors of interpretation may also enter the literature if researchers are so attached to a certain world view that they try to force both their own and others' results to fit that view. Such researchers tend to interpret an association as being causal on loose grounds, and they often give too much weight to "significant" p-values. They may also leave positive confounding or other bias uncontrolled and unmentioned. What is even worse, several cases of fraud, that is, fabrication of falsified results, have been revealed in science, to my knowledge at least once in occupational medicine. Although fraud is usually disclosed sooner or later, fraudulent scientists can cause much confusion first.

False Negative Results

The definition of safe work conditions is an important goal in occupational health research. Consequently, studies that convincingly demonstrate the absence of effect are at least as important as those revealing a harmful effect of an exposure. The problem is that the requirements for considering a study as convincingly negative are strict indeed. There is a fundamental difference between a true negative and a "non-positive" result.

Mathematically, proving a negative would require an infinite number of observations. In practice, it can never be achieved, so "infinite" must be exchanged for "large." A true negative study must therefore be *large*. In addition, it must be *sensitive* so that it can indeed detect an effect if there is one. Moreover, it must provide *accurate exposure data* because a study can be negative only with respect to prevailing or lower exposure levels. Of course, it must also otherwise be well designed and correctly executed, and its objective must be explicitly defined. Is the aim to exclude the risk of only one disease (e.g., cancer), or is it to assure complete safety of the studied conditions (if complete safety exists, which is doubtful)?

A true negative study must be large and sensitive, and it must have accurate exposure data.

A small negative study is better referred to as "non-positive," but it could equally well be named "uninformative" or "inconclusive." Nonpositive studies are generally small or medium-sized studies having an $\widehat{RR}$ near unity. The point estimate of the RR may even be clearly below 1, but as long as the confidence interval is wide and its upper bound is well above 1, the result is inconclusive rather than negative. Likewise, studies with a moderately elevated $\widehat{RR}$ may also be classified as nonpositive, if the lower bound of the confidence interval is below 1. In conventional jargon such a result would be called statistically nonsignificant. Such studies can, in a quantitative sense, rule out accentuated risks, or those in excess of the upper limit of the confidence interval.

Of course the terms "large" and "small" are vague terms. If "large" is defined as *many exposed cases* or a *large expected number*, the concept becomes somewhat less diffuse. Then "large" does not only mean that the number of subjects or person-years is large, but also that the disease is common in the study base. Together these properties result in many exposed cases. A case-referent design is similar in this respect because, if the case series is large and the exposure common, there will also be many exposed cases. The point is that it is not only the size of the cohort, or the number of cases in a case-referent study, that determines the size of the study. The frequency of the phenomenon of interest is also important. For example, the follow-up of a very large cohort, say half a million person-years, can be a small study base if the disease is rare.

Although somewhat alleviated, the problem is not solved by qualifying "large" as many exposed cases. The next question is, how many are "many"? Again no precise answer can be given. Qualitative studies need fewer cases than quantitative ones in order to be "large." One also has to be pragmatic. If either the disease or the exposure is rare, in general (e.g., angiosarcoma of the liver, exposure to beryllium), one must have less strict criteria for "large," perhaps 40 to 50 exposed cases. If, on the other hand, common phenomena are being studied (e.g., exposure to man-made mineral fibers, bronchial carcinoma), one could well require 200 or even more exposed cases in order to consider the study as "large." These figures are arbitrary and subjective, however, and other epidemiologists may choose other numbers.

Insensitive studies are characterized by a crude design (e.g., register linkage studies) and/or crude methods (e.g., occupational titles as surrogates for exposure). Insensitive studies are weak for the purpose of providing evidence in favor of the absence of an effect. They can be compared with an insensitive diagnostic clinical examination, such as a plain radiological examination for the diagnosis of a prolapsed lumbar disc. Such studies cannot prove that a certain exposure is without effect.

Negative studies can be related only to prevailing or lower exposure conditions, never to higher or longer exposures. This is a particularistic requirement, but, nevertheless, it is important from a practical point of view. In toxicology, most dose–response relationships have a threshold, and defining that threshold has an important practical application in the setting of hygienic standards. However, showing convincingly that no effect occurs under certain exposure conditions requires those conditions to be well characterized in quantitative terms. Unfortunately, such data are not easy to produce, at least not in retrospect, and this problem has ruined many otherwise valuable studies.

These considerations illustrate the difficulties facing researchers investigating a constellation in which no effect really exists. The demands on convincingly negative results are high indeed. No wonder that truly negative studies are rare in the literature. Therefore, the conclusion that some exposure is devoid of harmful effect (e.g., a certain chemical is *not* carcinogenic) must be based on a synthesis of the whole available literature; it can never rely on one single study. Hence all the scientific evidence (i.e., theoretical, experimental, and epidemiologic) that exists must be combined. Even so, a negative conclusion may be difficult to reach. For example, an expert group convened by the International Agency for Research on Cancer (IARC) could classify only one single chemical (caprolactam) as being probably noncarcinogenic out of the more than 700 agents reviewed.[3] The "negative" evidence for all the other agents lacking "positive" evidence was considered as insufficient.

Lack of Power

As pointed out earlier, dichotomizing studies into either positive or negative (and nonpositive) is artificial and wrong. When negativity is a function of the statistical power (size of the study), the positivity/negativity scale is a continuum. A nonpositive result due to low statistical power can exclude a risk higher than the upper limit of the confidence interval of the $\widehat{RR}$, of course in relation to prevailing exposure conditions and on the assumption that no negative bias or random error exists (see Chapter 5).

> *Example 4.* Suppose that the $\widehat{RR}$ for bronchial asthma is 1.75 in a group of 50 workers, as compared to 50 referents. Let the CI_{90} for the $\widehat{RR}$ be 0.68--4.54. The only thing that can be said is that the exposure prevailing in the study does not cause more than a fivefold increase of the risk to incur asthma. Such a result contains very little, if any, useful information.

Too small a study size can cause a true effect to pass undetected. This type II error is inversely proportional to the statistical power. Those with insight into epidemiology can easily spot a weakness of this type, but those with less experience may misinterpret the lack of statistical significance as indication of true negativity. As already mentioned, even seemingly large materials can, in fact, be small. The key issue is to secure enough exposed cases, and in this pursuit the selection of correct study type is important. If the disease is rare, a large study base is needed. Then a sampling of the study base becomes the only workable option, and a case-referent design is necessary. If the exposure is rare, it is best to define the study base as a follow-up of those having that exposure, and use a cohort design. The occurrence of diseases with a short duration cannot be studied effectively by a cross-sectional design, which measures prevalence, not incidence.

Low power also ensues whenever the study focuses on *wrong categories* of workers. Here "wrong" means exposed categories with a low likelihood of incurring the disease, for example, young age groups. If only occupationally active workers are studied and retired workers are omitted from a cancer study for reasons of convenience, tracing them being costly, important information is lost. Then the "truth," which in fact may be positive, could appear to be negative. Therefore, one should be careful to select the study material so that the appropriate age categories are well represented. For example, asbestos-induced mesothelioma can often be found in a study on comparatively young persons, if exposure has started early, while the excess of bronchial carcinoma caused by the same exposure may be better demonstrated in older age groups (although the background rate—the denominator—may be so high among older people that the RR is lowered for that reason). In this example, both younger and older age groups are informative, and the study should span a wide age range.

Whenever the study is qualitative, that is, when causality is the issue, one should have strict admissibility criteria, excluding subjects with *short and/or low exposure* from the exposed category. Likewise, in a case-referent study, the criteria for classifying someone as exposed should also be strict. Uncertain exposure should best be classified as "unknown;" otherwise nondifferential misclassification will dilute the effect and thereby mask a true risk. On the other hand, if the study is quantitative (the qualitative aspects already being known), subjects with low and/or short exposure must be included. Otherwise there will be no information on these exposure categories. Such a material should *not* be analyzed as a homogeneous group, however. This dilemma once again illustrates the importance of clear distinction between qualitative and quantitative studies. A qualitative study should concentrate on heavily exposed subjects; a quantitative one should span a wide range of exposures.

A qualitative study should focus on heavily exposed subjects, while a quantitative study should examine several exposure intensities.

Whenever the follow-up time is *too short*, or when the *latency time is left without consideration* in the analysis of data from a study on a disease with a long latency (e.g., work-related cancer), a falsely negative result will also emerge. Neglecting the latency period weakens the power because the study base will then be diluted with a follow-up of a period during which the outcome under study is unlikely (person-years are computed before the work-related disease could have developed). If the follow-up is too short, fewer cases will also occur.

The long latency time is a difficult problem when occupational cancer is being studied (see Chapter 6). The demand for quick results is in conflict with the long time span needed for achieving enough statistical power. However, the pressure from decision-makers should not be allowed to provoke too hasty conclusions based on premature (usually nonpositive) results. If preliminary results are made public, it is the authors' duty to emphasize their preliminary nature. Sometimes early publication is motivated, and it has now become routine to update studies published too early (from a scientific point of view) at regular intervals. Early publication combined with later updating appears to be a satisfactory compromise, as long as the authors clearly explain the nature of each consecutive report.

Several different latency times should be tried in the analysis in order to identify when the maximal effect occurs, but this practice requires a sufficiently large material. Figure 1 illustrates schematically why cancer studies are uninformative during the first years of follow-up. The informativeness also decreases when the follow-up proceeds partly because the "background noise" increases and partly because the peak of work-induced cancer has already passed. The figure is oversimplified for pedagogic reasons, and all numbers are fictive. Moreover, the shape of the curve fits only for an initiator. It would be different for a promotor, or for a mixed initiator and promotor exposure.

Falsely negative conclusions may be reached when
• The study material is too small
• The study design is inefficient
• Wrong exposure categories are studied
• The exposure is too low and/or too short
• The follow-up is too short or incomplete
• Allowance is not made for a latency period

Fortunately, neglecting such elementary requirements of study design is now less prevalent than some years ago. Moreover, crudely wrong interpretations of data rarely pass the publishing threshold of good journals. However, such reports may be published in mediocre scientific journals without strict peer review, and poor papers can still be read at scientific congresses with lax or no advance review of the abstracts.

Lack of statistical power is not the only reason why a study may fail to detect an existing effect. There are also other causes; some of them are discussed in the following sections.

Insensitivity

The use of *crude indicators*, be it for the disease or for the exposure, masks

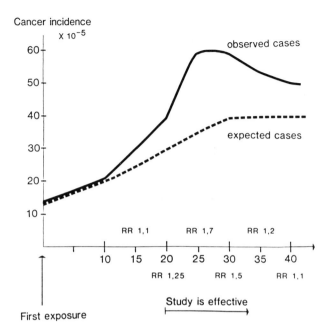

Figure 1. Simplified example showing the importance of accounting for the latency time in studies of work-related cancers. The study can detect effects only when a sufficiently long period of time has elapsed. Later the high background incidence masks the effect.

true effects. Especially when the objective is to document the absence of all kinds of effects, say, for the purpose of setting hygienic standards, the study must be sensitive. For example, mortality is too crude an indicator when the objective is to exclude all types of health effects. Nevertheless, mere lack of increased mortality in a study is frequently interpreted as indicative of safety. This conclusion is particularly doubtful when the comparison is made with reference to national or even regional general mortality statistics.

Random errors tend to mask existing differences. They occur when the measurements are poorly standardized, when their precision is low, and when the indicators are crude. Random errors have been discussed in Chapter 5 and are therefore not treated in this context.

Table 1. Effect of a 10% Nondifferential Misclassification on the Point Estimate of the OR. Correct OR = (40:60)/(10:90) = 6.0; Incorrect OR = (42:58)/(18:82) = 3.3.

Correct Classification		10% Misclassification
Cases		
Exposed	40	36 True positives
		4 False negatives
Unexposed	60	54 True negatives
		6 False positives
Referents		
Exposed	10	9 True positives
		1 False negative
Unexposed	90	81 True negatives
		9 False positives

Misclassification

The powerful effect-masking consequence of nondifferential misclassification was not fully appreciated until recently. The direction of the error of the $\widehat{RR}$, arising from such misclassification, is toward unity (i.e., masking a true effect, be it etiologic or preventive). Even a minor nondifferential misclassification produces a substantial negative error.

Example 5. Suppose, in a case-referent study, that 40 cases out of 100 and 10 referents out of 100 are found to have been exposed to a particular chemical. The correct estimate of the OR is then (40:60)/(10:90) = 6.0. Suppose there is a 10% nondifferential misclassification (i.e., every tenth subject is classified wrongly). Table 1 shows what happens.

This example shows how strong the masking effect of a relatively minor misclassification can be. A 20% error would drop the $\widehat{OR}$ to 2.2 and a 50% error to 1.

Often the correctness of past exposure data is difficult to ascertain, and nondifferential misclassification cannot be avoided. One can only speculate about the number of false negative results that have arisen from such misclassification. Studies in which occupational titles are used as proxies of exposure are often deemed a priori to remain uninformative for reasons of misclassification when the effect of a specific exposure is being studied.

Miscellaneous Errors

Sometimes the measures of disease chosen by the researchers may be *inappropriate* or *irrelevant* for the purpose of revealing effects of an exposure.

Example 6. Some years ago a study was published, in which lead workers with present or 5-year mean blood lead levels of 60—80 µg/100 mL (2.89—3.86 µmol/L) were compared to those with levels below 60 µg/100 mL (2.89 µmol/L).[7] Many biochemical and other indicators of illness were measured, among them no less than 29 biochemical laboratory tests. No statistically significant differences were found between the groups. The authors concluded that "there were no significant differences in the health of workers with blood lead concentrations between 60 and 80 µg/dL." They also stated: "It is our opinion that the current [in 1978] blood lead standard of 80 µg/dL can be kept, unless more data will support the OSHA proposal."

A very remarkable flaw in this study was that no tests whatsoever measuring disturbances of the protoporphyrin synthesis were included and that there were no measurements of neurophysiological or psychological functions. Making a *general* negative statement without the study of these parameters, which are generally known to be the critical (most sensitive) effects of lead toxicity, represents severe misinterpretation of toxicologic and epidemiologic data. In addition to basing the statement on wrong indicators of effect, the authors can be criticized for using too small contrasts; dichotomizing at 60 µg/100 mL instead of using an occupationally unexposed reference group substantially decreases the sensitivity of the study.

Falsely negative conclusions can also be reached when
- ## The measures of morbidity are crude
- ## There are random errors
- ## Nondifferential misclassification occurs
- ## Wrong or irrelevant morbidity indicators are used

Finally, *systematic errors* can also cause false negative results. Negative confounding probably occurs as often as positive confounding, although the latter has received more attention. Misclassification can also be differential or systematic, for example, if exposure is systematically underestimated for the cases as compared to the referents. This is a possibility when fatal diseases are being studied and the referents are drawn as a sample from the study base. In such a situation, the exposure history will predominantly be gathered from close relatives of the cases, but more often from the (alive) referents themselves. The subjects themselves remember the work history better than close relatives do; therefore seemingly more positive exposure histories may be obtained for the referents than the cases and result in the masking of the true effect as a consequence of systematic misclassification. Perhaps the best known negative systematic error is the healthy worker effect (Chapter 5). Negative bias is also frequent in cross-sectional studies because of health-based selection out from the exposed job.

SUPPORTING EVIDENCE FOR CAUSE-EFFECT INFERENCES

When systematic errors or random variation has been judged to be unlikely explanations for an observed association between two phenomena, the time has come to evaluate whether the association is causal or only a so-called statistical association. As stated several times before, nonexperimental research is weaker than experiments in supporting causality. Therefore, the scientific inference that one phenomenon causes another must utilize *all available knowledge*, not only the results of a single study, not only epidemiologic research, and not any isolated observation alone. In 1965, Sir Austin Bradford Hill[2] formulated nine general criteria for the judgment of causality. These criteria have become classic even though their applicability in epidemiology has been criticized recently (e.g., References 8 and 9). In spite of the doubts raised, Hill's criteria deserve consideration, and they are listed here together with their most pertinent counterarguments.

1. *Strong association.* The stronger the association, that is, the higher and more stable the $\widehat{RR}$, the more credible the causality. Small studies are an exception, as discussed before. However, a weak association does not rule out causality. For example, the exposure may have been low, or the study may have been diluted by random errors.

2. *Consistent evidence.* The consistency of evidence speaks in favor of causality. Hill stated that if the same association has been found by many researchers, and under different circumstances, causality is probable. The counterargument is that the studies may have been done with different methodology and that some of them may be better than others. Furthermore, if the causal agent needs complementary causes to become operative, they may not always be present. Hence lack of consistency does not rule out causality, although its presence speaks in favor of it.

3. *Specificity of the association.* Hill stated that, if an association is confined to certain groups of workers who have well-defined exposure conditions and who exhibit the same morbidity pattern, causality gains credibility. This criterion is definitely wrong. There are many single causes that can cause different diseases (e.g., smoking that causes many types of cancer, coronary heart disease, bronchitis, etc., arsenic that causes both lung and skin cancer as well as coronary heart disease, carbon disulfide that causes coronary heart disease, cerebrovascular disease, and neurological diseases, etc.).

4. *Temporality.* The cause must precede the effect. Whenever the disease breaks out soon after exposure, the relationship is straightforward. If the disease has a long latency, the exposure must have occurred early enough for the disease to have time to develop. Everyone agrees that this requirement is necessary, although it is, at times, difficult to verify.

5. *Biological gradient.* There should be evidence of a dose–response relationship. However, confounding factors cannot be separated from such a relation. Moreover, if the effect is maximal in a study (i.e., everybody gets the disease, as has been seen for erionite exposure and mesothelioma), the study cannot demonstrate a dose–response relationship.

6. *Biological plausibility.* The fact that the finding is biologically plausible speaks in favor of causality. The relation between such plausibility and causality is strongly inferred in Bayesian thinking, as discussed earlier in this chapter. However, Pott could not explain why chimney sweeps incurred scrotal cancer from their work, and yet he was correct in his assumption that the disease was work-related. The fact that biological mechanisms are still unknown to scientists does not influence scientific truths.

7. *Coherence of evidence.* According to Hill, if experimental work and theory support an epidemiologic finding, the evidence for causality is corroborated. However, it is not quite clear how coherence differs from plausibility. Perhaps the distinction is that there should not be conflicting evidence.
8. *Experimental evidence.* Human beings can rarely be experimentally exposed, and extrapolation from animal experiments is problematic. Even so, if the same effect that has been observed in an epidemiologic study can be induced in animal experiments, the causality of the association gains credibility. Likewise, a change in exposure that is followed by a change in morbidity supports causality. The weight given the effects of actively changing exposure has to do with the similarities between experimental research and interventive epidemiology. Unfortunately, only few intervention studies have been published in the epidemiologic literature on occupational medicine.
9. *Analogy.* Reasoning by analogy can help judge causality. For example, if a certain chemical is a known carcinogen and a related compound shows an association with cancer in an epidemiologic study, the causality is easier to accept than if the two substances were unrelated. Unfortunately, with good imagination, one can find analogies nearly everywhere.

It is important that all available scientific evidence be utilized when the causality of an epidemiologic association is judged. In spite of all attempts to construct guidelines for evaluating causality, this process is still predominantly subjective, and those who know most of the subject matter, and who understand the rules of scientific inference best, are the most likely to be correct. But even authorities, as all humans, can be mistaken, a fact that is well known from the history of science.

Hill never meant his criteria to be absolute rules. On the contrary, he stated that no "hard-and-fast" rules can be given for causal inference. A symposium was recently held on the topic of causal inference, and the divergent views expressed clearly showed that causal inference is no simple matter. The proceedings[9] are recommended as further reading for those interested in more in-depth considerations of this central and interesting topic.

The purpose of this chapter has been to explain to readers how difficult it is to interpret epidemiologic articles. In general, epidemiologic methods are too crude to reveal slight risks. Most of the errors affecting cohort and cross-sectional studies have a negative direction, and the same is true for some of the errors of case-referent studies. Until now, most of the efforts of researchers have been devoted to controlling positive bias, and those of the readers' to revealing such errors. So-called conservative risk assessments have been considered indicative of sound judgment, while less conservative interpretations have been thought of as uncritical. In my view, one should realize the effect of the crudeness of epidemiology in risk assessment. Crude studies and too conservative an interpretation can, alone or in combination, easily lead to real hazards being overlooked, that is, to the *underestimation of risk*. Underestimation can have serious consequences for those involved, both exposed workers and the public at large.

REFERENCES

1. Bourbonnais, R., F. Meyer, and G. Theriault. "Validity of self reported work history," *Br. J. Ind. Med.* 45:29 (1988).
2. Hill, A. B. "The environment and disease: association or causation?" *Proc. R. Soc. Med.* 58:1217 (1965).
3. IARC. "Monographs on the Evaluation of Carcinogenic Risks to Humans, Suppl 7." Overall evaluations of carcinogenicity: an updating of IARC monographs volumes 1 to 42. (Lyon: IARC, 1987).
4. Kurppa, K., S. Tola, S. Hernberg, and M. Tolonen. "Industrial solvents and the liver," *Lancet* 1:129 (1983).
5. Miettinen, O. S. *Theoretical Epidemiology: Principles of Occurrence Research in Medicine* (New York: John Wiley & Sons, 1985).
6. Nurminen, T., and K. Kurppa. "Office employment, work with video display terminals, and course of pregnancy," *Scand. J. Work Environ. Health* 14:293 (1988).
7. Ramirez-Cervantes, B., J. W. Embree, C. H. Hine, K. W. Nelson, M. O. Vernes, and R. D. Putnam. "Health assessment of employees with different body burdens of lead," *J. Occup. Med.* 20:610 (1978).
8. Rothman, K. J. *Modern Epidemiology* (Boston, MA: Little Brown, 1986).
9. Rothman, K. J. *Causal Inference* (Boston, MA: Epidemiology Resources, 1988).
10. Rothman, K. J. "No adjustments are needed for multiple comparisons," *Epidemiology* 1:43 (1990).
11. Sotaniemi, E. A., Seppo Sutinen, Sirkka Sutinen, A. J. Arranto, and O. Pelkonen. "Liver injury in subjects occupationally exposed to chemicals in low doses," *Acta Med. Scand.* 212:207 (1982).

Index